Cooking Well

Honey for Health & Beauty

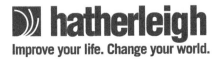

hatherleigh

Improve your life. Change your world.

About the *Cooking Well* series

We have long known that proper nutrition plays an important role in guarding health and preventing the onset of disease. The *Cooking Well* series was created to help you learn more about the important role of nutrient-rich meals when living with your particular disorder. With *Cooking Well*, you will discover that there are many enjoyable ways to prepare delightful, great-tasting meals that are packed with a variety of healthful benefits.

Hatherleigh has a long history of providing our readers with books that help people improve their lives, whether through exercise, nutrition, or mental well-being. We are pleased to share with you the message of good health in the *Cooking Well* series.

HONEY FOR HEALTH & BEAUTY

Text copyright © 2009 Hatherleigh Press, Ltd.

Hatherleigh Press is committed to preserving and protecting the natural resources of the Earth. Environmentally responsible and sustainable practices are embraced within the company's mission statement.

Hatherleigh Press is a member of the Publishers Earth Alliance, committed to preserving and protecting the natural resources of the planet while developing a sustainable business model for the book publishing industry.

www.hatherleighpress.com

DISCLAIMER
This book offers healthy eating suggestions for educational purposes only. In no case should it be a substitute for, nor replace, a healthcare professional. Consult your healthcare professional before starting any new diet.

Library of Congress Cataloging-in-Publication Data is available upon request
ISBN: 978-1-57826-288-5

All Hatherleigh Press titles are available for bulk purchase, special promotions, and premiums. For information about reselling and special purchase opportunities, please call 1-800-528-2550 and ask for the Special Sales Manager.

Interior design by Nick Macagnone
Photos by Catarina Astrom
10 9 8 7 6

Special thanks to the National Honey Board, whose informative and helpful web site provided the content for much of this book.

Printed in the United States of America

Dedication

This book is dedicated to the humble and hard working honey bee, without which we could not survive

Table of Contents

Foreword

"Honey" is a lifelong love affair in my family. It represents "a Lune de Miel" that started when I was a young girl.

I remember my grand-mother serving us toasts with this beautiful gold color honey for breakfast. She would tell us that it is good for our health, growth, and not as bad as white sugar on our teeth. My uncle also used to bring us the most delicious honey from his favorite farms. He would tell us stories about the bees and would teach us about the different flavors of honey. My dad would bring home this thick rich creamy honey that I could eat by the spoonful! And let's not forget that soothing hot milk and honey for my sore throat. Today, I favor tea with honey.

I've also come to realize that honey had many other health benefits and even therapeutic properties. Honey has been described as "Gods' Nectar" and it is certainly magical to me. It excites and pleasures my taste buds like no other sugar. But such a delectable experience can only be lived with the finest, most natural honey. You need to educate yourself and your palate just as you would with wine. Color, concentration, viscosity, aroma, taste, finish, and complexity are the most important elements in defining the best honey. Flowers or plants varieties, the region, and the manufacturing process will differentiate many honeys from each other. Try as many as you can, you will learn to appreciate their uniqueness.

By the way, did you know that honey mixed with olive oil, lemon juice, and lavender makes a great facial mask? Try it sometime!

Chef Marie-Annick Courtier

Introduction

In *Honey for Health & Beauty* the long misunderstood bee has now, at last, received its well deserved place as queen in the animal kingdom.

As a physician and a homeopath, the use of honey for medical treatments is well known to me. From a medicinal healing agent and culinary nectar to an anti-wrinkle beauty product, honey has nourished and brought aid to humankind for many generations. The uses of honey abound, and, with this book, honey formulas and recipes are no longer old wives' tales. Readers will be delighted with the fascinating facts about honey and honey bees, as well as the delicious recipes and beauty treatments.

In addition to providing practical information, this book provides some of the latest results from scientific studies. The honeybee is the source for an amazing product, and the possibilities of honey use for health are finally being backed up by medical science—studies around the world are revealing the power of honey as a natural "wonderdrug." *Honey for Health & Beauty* discusses, citing the latest research from the National Honey Board website, scientifically sound examples that present the possibilities of using honey for variety of health remedies—as a replacement for a carbohydrate energy booster when exercising, as a prebiotic, as an aid in calcium absorption, as an antimicrobial, and as help in managing chronic conditions, among other things. As a physician, I have been aware of the broad spectrum of antibacterial effects of honey and have used it extensively for such conditions as sore throats. Now, anyone can use honey with confidence.

Honey is also a delicious, nutritious sugar substitute. Not only is it perfect for sweet recipes, like desserts, but with its unique, rich flavor, honey can also enhance main dishes featuring fish and meat, as well as vegetarian stir fry and salads. Using honey in a wide variety of recipes may allow us to tap into its powers as a regulator of "friendly bacteria" at the same time that we enjoy its delightful flavor.

After reading *Honey for Health & Beauty*, I am now enthusiastic to increase the use of honey in some of my favorite dishes, as well as a healing agent.

As honey has been appreciated by many, so will this book.

Lauren Feder, M.D.
Author: *Natural Baby and Childcare,*
The Parents' Concise Guide to Vaccinations

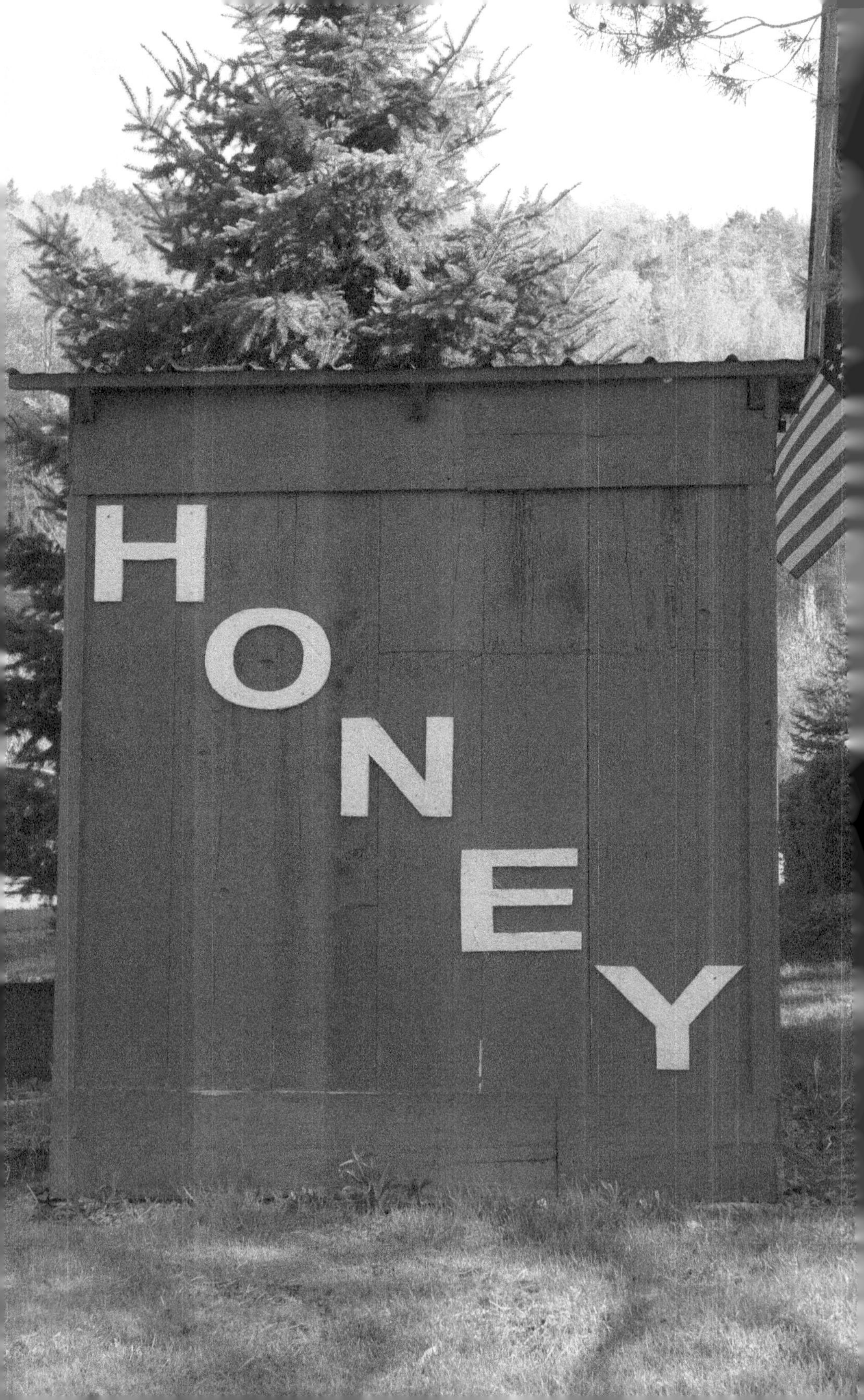
HONEY

Chapter 1

The Story of Honey

Before honey arrives on your kitchen table, it has been part of a remarkable process and quite a journey. In order to produce one jar of honey, bees travel a distance roughly of 500,000 miles. That's the equivalent of a round-trip to the moon! But it's all just another day's work for the diligent honey bee, nature's powerhouse insect.

What is honey? Honey is actually flower nectar that has been consumed, regurgitated, and rehydrated by bees until it reaches the perfect consistency. Beeswax, which is used to build the beehive, is also the product of nectar. A honeybee has to log a lot of miles, traveling from flower to flower, to accumulate enough nectar to create honey. Once a honeybee gathers nectar, it returns to the beehive and begins to process what will become honey. In the hive, honey is stored in six-sided hexagonal chambers. The honeycomb structure of the hive is also ideal for use as "rooms" for the queen bee to lay her eggs.

Honey is mostly made up of fructose, glucose, and water. It also contains a variety of other sugars, and trace amounts of enzymes, minerals vitamins and amino acids.

In order for honey to be gathered for human consumption, the honey-covered walls of the hive are removed and placed in a spinner. Rotating rapidly, the spinner separates the liquid from the comb.

Besides being honey-producers, honeybees help put fresh fruits and vegetables on your table, and ensure that our fields and woods are lush and healthy. How? When they gather nectar from flowers, honeybees perform pollination. Pollination is the process where, through the transfer of pollen from one plant to another.

Honey bees pollinate 80% of the fresh fruits and vegetables we eat.

Forms of Honey

Although most of us may only be familiar with one type of honey, liquid honey, there are actually many different forms of honey available for human consumption. In addition to being offered as a golden liquid, honey can also be found in the following forms:

- **Comb honey** is attached to the comb from the hive. The comb can be eaten along with the honey.
- Cut comb is **liquid honey** that contains chunks of the honey comb. This is also known as liquid-cut comb combination.
- **Liquid honey** is the most popular and widely known type of honey. This is honey is clear and pure and doesn't contain any visible crystals. Liquid honey is the most convenient type of honey for use in baking.
- Naturally **crystallized honey** is liquid honey that has crystallized because the glucose (sugar) content of the honey has separated from the liquid. This is a natural process.
- **Whipped** or **creamed honey** has been intentionally crystallized during manufacture and carefully blended so that the resulting honey is thick yet spreadable, much like butter. In many countries around the world, whipped honey is the honey of choice.

It takes nectar from about 2 million flowers to create 1 pound of honey.

In her lifetime, the average honeybee will make produce only one-twelfth of a teaspoon of honey.

A queen bee can lay up to 3,000 eggs in one day— that's 175-200,000 per year.

Communication is key for honeybees, who must be able to tell each other the location of flowers, their invaluable source of nectar. Honeybees communicate using a series of movements similar to dancing, called the "waggle dance."

Variety is the Spice of Life: Honey Variety

In addition to the different types of honey to choose from, there are also a variety of honey colors and flavors available. Honey color ranges from a very pale yellow that is nearly colorless, to dark brown. As for flavor, the taste of honey can be mild or intense; some types of honey even taste like the flower they came from, such as orange blossom honey. The color and flavor of honey varies widely depending on the source of the nectar—that is, depending on what flower the honey visited to gather the nectar and make the honey.

> **In the United States alone there are over 300 kinds of honey.**

There are several types of honey available all over the world. The most common types of honey, and the flowers that produce the nectar for the honey, include:

- ❀ **Alfalfa** is a legume with blue flowers found most commonly in Utah, Nevada, Idaho, Oregon and a majority of the western states. Alfalfa honey is pale amber and has a delicate flavor, making it the perfect accompaniment for a variety of foods.
- ❀ **Avocado honey** is gathered from the avocado blossom. Avocado honey most often comes from California. Dark in color, avocado honey tastes rich and has a thick, buttery consistency.
- ❀ **Basswood** is a tree with cream-colored blooms. This honey is found in areas from Southern Canada, to Alabama and down to Texas appears white.
- ❀ The **blueberry** bush produces tiny white flowers whose nectar helps the bees produce a full-flavored honey that is light amber in color. This honey is commonly produced in New England and Michigan.
- ❀ **Buckwheat** plants bloom early in the season in climates that are cool and moist. These plants produce honey that is dark in color and has a distinctive flavor.
- ❀ **Clover plants** are the most popular honey plants in the U.S. Types of clover used to produce clover honey include white clover, alsike clover, and white and yellow sweet clover. Clover honey has a mild and delicate flavor and can appear white or extra light amber, depending on its source.
- ❀ The **Eucalyptus** plant has over 500 species and many hybrids. Generally, eucalyptus honey has a bold taste that some describe as being slightly medicinal.

- **Fireweed** is a herb that grows in the open woods and is most commonly found in the Northern and Pacific States as well as Canada. Fireweed is easy to spot—it grows from 3 to 5 feet tall and has lovely pink flowers. Fireweed honey is light in color.
- The **orange** tree produces white blossoms and is a common source of honey in Florida, Texas, Arizona, and California. Orange blossom honey comes from a variety of citrus sources, and is extra light amber in color. It has a distinctive taste with a hint of orange flavor.
- **Sage** shrubs can be found along with California coast and in the Sierra Nevada mountains. Sage honey has a mild taste and appears white.
- **Sourwood** trees are found in the Appalachian mountains. Sourwood honey has a pleasant sweet flavor that is also spicy and similar to anise (which has a flavor similar to licorice).
- The **tulip polar** is a tree with large greenish-yellow flowers. Tulip poplar honey is produced from southern New England to southern Michigan and south to the Gulf states east of the Mississippi. The honey is dark amber in color, yet its flavor is more delicate that most dark honeys.
- **Tupelo** trees have clusters of flowers which later develop into soft fruit. Tupelo honey is the leading type of honey is southern Georgia and northwestern Florida. Tupelo honey is white or extra light amber in color and has a subtle, pleasant flavor. Tupelo honey will not granulate.

For more details on these and more floral sources, and to locate specific varieties of honey, visit *www.honeylocator.com*.

> **Sidr honey, which is harvested only twice a year from bees that feed exclusively on the pollen of the Sidr tree in the Hadramaut Mountains of Eastern Yemen, is said to be the most expensive honey in the world. It is priced at $200 per kilogram! Sidr honey is prized by many for its medicinal benefits as well as its rich, remarkable taste.**

Honey in Your Home

With such a wide variety of delicious honeys to choose from, you may want to have many flavors in your home to try in tea, on toast, or just by the spoonful. When using honey for baking and cooking, however, it is generally advisable to choose a honey with a mild flavor, so it does not overpower your dish. Keep in mind, though, that as you continue to experiment with honey in your dishes, you can feel free to try different honey flavors.

Honey Storage Tips

Here are some tips for honey storage.

✿ Honey should be stored at room temperature. The kitchen counter or a pantry shelf are perfectly suitable.

✿ If you refrigerate honey, you'll notice that it will crystallize and separate rather quickly. This is a natural process and it does not mean the honey is ruined. In fact, it is easy to get honey back to its smooth, liquid state. If your honey crystallizes, heat water until warm in a pot large enough for your honey jar. Then, place the honey in its glass jar, in the water and stir the honey until the crystals dissolve. Or, you can place the honey, with the lid off, in a microwave-safe container for 30 seconds. Stir after 30 seconds and if there are still crystals present, microwave for another 30 seconds and stir. Continue this process until the crystals dissolve. Take care not to boil or scorch the honey.

✿ Remarkably enough, honey stored in a sealed container is edible even after several years. However, honey will lose its flavor and delicate aroma over time, so it is generally recommended that honey be discarded after two years in order to ensure best taste.

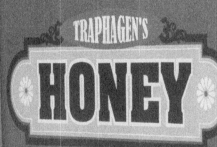

Chapter 2

Honey, Health and Healing

Most of us know honey as a delicious sweet treat that can enhance a variety of dishes and beverages (see page [tk] for some delicious recipe ideas). Yet you may not be aware that honey also has key qualities that make this amber liquid a healthful, all-natural nutrition supplement. Furthermore, modern medicine has recently conducted studies that point to ways in which honey can actually heal several diseases and ailments.

Honey and Health: Nutrient Content

Honey is primarily made up of fructose, glucose, and water. Honey also contains small amounts of several vitamins and minerals, including niacin, riboflavin, pantothenic acid, calcium, copper, iron, magnesium, manganese, phosphorus, potassium and zinc. There are also characteristics to honey that make it act as an antioxidant.

An antioxidant is a molecule that slows or stops oxidation, a chemical reaction that can produce free radicals. Free radicals are highly-reactive elements that can damage cells and, it is speculated, lead to conditions such as cancer, cardiovascular disease, Parkinson's, and Alzheimer's. Antioxidant-rich foods may help prevent cellular damage and protect against the development of numerous diseases. This is why a diet high in antioxidant-rich fruits and vegetables is recommended by doctors and nutritionists alike.

Liquid honey is about 1 to 1½ times sweeter tasting than sugar, yet it has a lower calorie content.

Recent research indicates that honey's antioxidant capacity can be just as effective as the antioxidants in some fruits and vegetables.

Currently, the antioxidant capacity of honey is thought to be the result of several compounds acting together, including phenolics, peptides, organic acids, and enzymes. In the article "Chronic honey consumption increases plasma antioxidant concentration", Dr. Gross found that regular consumption of several tablespoons of honey over a 29-day period increased antioxidant levels in healthy adult subjects. Additionally, an article published in the American Dietetic Association revealed that simply substituting honey for sugar can lead to an increase in antioxidants that is equivalent of eating a handful of antioxidant rich berries or nuts. Choosing honey to specifically sweeten black tea has also been shown to increase the presence of antioxidants in the body. In summary, numerous reports suggest that consuming honey on a regular basis, or at least substituting honey for sugar, can greatly increase the body's antioxidant level and help protect against free radicals. Making honey a part of your diet is an easy way to strengthen your body's defense system.

> **The amount and type of antioxidants in honey depends on the flower that is the honey's source. Generally, darker honeys (such as buckwheat honey) are richer in antioxidants than lighter honeys.**

Honey as a Prebiotic

Our gastrointestinal tract contains many types of "good bacteria" that help to regulate digestion and ensure good health. One type of good bacteria is called bifidobacteria. Research has shown that one way to increase the presence of bifidobacteria is to consume foods containing prebiotics, which help the good bacteria to replicate and grow. Honey contains a variety of substances that can act as a prebiotic and encourage the growth of good bacteria. In one recent study, scientists at Michigan State University found that adding honey to yogurt can increase the efficacy of good bacteria.

Honey and Calcium Absorption

Honey itself is not a source of calcium, but researchers at Purdue University have found that consuming honey helps calcium from other dietary sources to be more easily absorbed in the body. Although more research is needed, the possibility that honey may aid in calcium absorption makes it an appealing addition to dishes featuring sources of calcium like milk, yogurt, and cheese.

Honey and Athletics

With a carbohydrate content of 17 grams per tablespoon, honey is a good source of carbohydrates, which provide quick, natural energy for athletes or anyone on the go who needs a healthy boost. Is well-known among athletes that consuming carbs before, after, and during exercise helps muscles recover from intense activity, prevent premature fatigue, and improve overall performance. In the article Honey can serve as an effective carbohydrate replacement during exercise, researchers found that honey was just as effective as a sugar mixture in increasing endurance for nine male endurance athletes. These results suggest that honey may serve as an inexpensive alternative to sports gels. For the non-athlete, the quick, nutrient-rich boost that honey provides is a healthy alternative to caffeine or sugary candy bars that anyone can feel good about (see page 111 for a great-tasting and nutritious energy bar recipe featuring honey).

Honey and Healing

For centuries, cultures all around the world have used honey to guard health and cure illness, as well as a sweetener. Through the ages, honey has been a "cure-all" for just about everything, from complaints like sleeplessness and indigestion to serious conditions like wounds. As unusual as this may sound to us, science has recently discovered that these ancient medical doctors may have been onto something: results have shown that many of honey's properties can indeed be used to cure a wide range of diseases inside and outside the body. These conditions include wounds and burns, as well as internal ailments such as coughs and sore throat.

> One type of honey known to be particularly rich in antioxidants is Manuka honey, produced in New Zealand from the Manuka bush. The Manuka bush is more commonly known as the tea tree plant.

Honey and Healing: Recent Studies

The studies below present a brief overview of the ways in which honey has worked to cure a number of ailments and why this golden liquid has proved promising as a treatment.

Honey as an Antimicrobial

Honey's "miracle cure" quality is due largely in part to its role as an antimicrobial agent. Antimicrobial means that honey helps to kill harmful bacteria without damaging fragile tissue. Recently, research into the abilities of honey as an antimicrobial agent capable of killing bacteria has increased due to the rise in "superbugs". Superbugs are illnesses caused by strains of bacteria that are resistant to antibiotics. In some cases, without the aid of conventional treatment, these superbugs can be fatal.

In the article "The sensitivity to honey of Gram-positive cocci of clinical significance isolated from wounds" Dr.'s Cooper, Molan and Harding described how honey can be useful in treating wounds unable to heal because they are infected with antibiotic-resistant bacteria. The study found that, when three types of antibiotic-resistent bacteria (methicillin-resistant Staphylococcus aureus, MRSA; vancomyacin-sensitive enterococci, VSE; and vancomyacin-resistnant enterococci, VRE) were exposed to honey, that honey halted the growth of the harmful bacteria. This suggests that honey may be useful in treating wounds that resist conventional antibiotic treatment.

In another study "Local application of honey for treatment of neonatal postoperative wound infection", Dr. Vardi and his colleagues found that honey can also be effective in helping wounds to heal even in the most vulnerable of patients: infants. During this study, honey was used to treat open, infected wounds in nine infants who were recovering from surgery. The infants had been treated with antibiotics, but the wounds failed to heal. Dressings soaked in honey were applied to the wounds and changed twice daily. After five days of treatment, all infants showed improvement. After 21 days, the wounds had closed in all of the infants. There were no adverse reactions to the treatment with honey.

These results indicate that, with further research, honey could be an important treatment for individuals of any age who have wounds infected with antibiotic-resistant bacteria.

Honey as Treatment for Chronic Conditions

There has also been recent evidence suggesting that honey can be effective in managing certain conditions, similar to the way in which certain prescription drugs are used to manage diabetes, heart disease, and allergies. Although there is still a long way to go in this area of study, with the rising cost of health care, the potential of honey as a way to ensure long-term health for individuals afflicted or at risk for chronic conditions is promising.

In the article "Natural honey lowers plasma glucose, C-reactive protein, and blood lipids in healthy, diabetic, and hyperlipidaemic comparison with dextrose and sucrose", Dr. Al-Waili compared the increase in blood glucose levels in diabetics. One group of volunteers was fed honey, and the other group was given a sugar mixture. When blood glucose levels were measured, Dr. Al-Waili found that the level of blood sugar in the body was lower in the patients who had consumed honey. In another study, "Natural honey lowers plasma prostaglandin concentrations in normal individuals", Dr. Al-Waili found that when twelve healthy individuals consumed natural unprocessed honey with water once a day for 15 days, that the concentration of prostaglandins in their bloodstream was reduced. Although further studies like these are needed, results like this suggest that consuming honey may keep blood glucose levels low, resulting in a lower risk of heart disease for some patients.

Honey and Oral Health

Honey has been known to prevent the growth of a variety of bacteria, including bacteria in the mouth.

In the article "Antioxidant and Antimicrobial Activity of Honeys Against Oral Pathogens" several types of honey were tested (including sage, orange, tupelo, and manuka honey) and it was found that all were found effective in halting the growth of several bacteria, including porphoromonas gingivalus (otherwise known as gingivitis.)

In another promising study, "The effects of manuka honey on plaque and gingivitis: a pilot study", Dr. English and his colleagues evaluated the efficacy of Manuka honey in fighting dental plaque and gingivitis. For this study, Manuka honey was used to make a chewable form of honey called "honey leather," which can be chewed like a stick of gum. Thirty subjects were divided into two groups: 1 group chewed sugarless gum for 10 minutes, 3 times a day following meals, and the other group chewed the honey leather. At the end of the study, those who had chewed the honey product showed lower levels of plaque and lower occurrence of gingivitis symptoms. Those who had chewed gum showed no improvement in plaque or gingivitis reduction compared to if they had not chewed at all. These results suggest certain kinds of honey may be an effective way to prevent gingivitis and periodontal disease.

Honey and Cough Suppression

In the study titled "Effect of Honey, Dextromethorphan, and No Treatment on Nocturnal Cough and Sleep Quality for Coughing Children and Their Parents", researchers found that when children had two groups of ages 2-18 with a cough were given cough medicine DM and the other group was given a doest of buckwheat honey 30 minutes before bedtime, that the honey was just as effective in reducing the cough as the DM cough syrup. Honey was rated by the parents as most favorable for relieving cough and helping their children to sleep. In the future, some parents may decide to choose honey over DM since DM has been known to have questionable side effects.

Honey in the Medicine Cabinet

Although science is still a long way off from recommending treatment with honey in much the same way prescriptions and over the counter medicines are prescribed, there are many common household honey remedies that you can use with assurance. Here are a few ways you can take advantage of the natural healing benefits of honey in your home.

Honey Remedies

Before you try any honey remedies or recipes, keep in mind that honey should not be fed to infants younger than one year of age due to the possibility of a serious illness called botulism. Infant botulism is caused by bacterial spores. Although these spores may sound dangerous, they can in fact be found throughout our environment and in soil, dust, air, and in raw fruits and vegetables. These spores are routinely consumed without problems by children and adults. However, because infants lack a fully developed gastrointestinal tract, these spores can cause the disease known as botulism. While incidents of infant botulism caused by honey are rare, the Centers for Disease Control and Prevention, the American Academy of Pediatrics and the National Honey Board agree that the honey should not be fed to infants under one year of age.

> The use of honey and honey products for healing purposes is called apitherapy.

Because a sore throat could be the result of a wide variety of ailments, be sure to consult your doctor if you have a fever, or if symptoms continue for more than a few days.

Honey & Sore Throat

For decades, singers have used honey to soothe their throats before an important performance. But anyone can use honey to ease a sore throat.

Try a spoonful of honey as often as is needed for sore throat relief. Honey's slow-moving liquid quality will coat your throat and help relieve irritation.

You can also try the Honey Citrus Soother, below, for extra Vitamin C.

Honey Citrus Soother

serves 4

ingredients

3 tea bags green or black
1 cinnamon stick
3 cups boiling water
1/4 cup honey
1 cup grapefruit juice

cooking instructions

Place tea bags and cinnamon stick in a 1-quart tea pot. Add boiling water; steep 3 to 5 minutes. Remove cinnamon stick and tea bags; discard. Stir in grapefruit juice and honey.

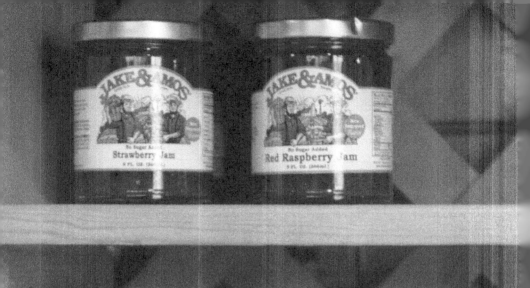

JAKE & AMOS

No Sugar Added
Strawberry Jam
8 FL OZ. (266ml.)

JAKE & AMOS

No Sugar Added
Red Raspberry Jam
8 FL OZ. (266ml.)

Traphagen's Honey
Route 23A West P.O. Box J
Hunter, N.Y. 12442   518-263-4150

PURE . NATURAL . HONEY

NET WT. 2 LBS.

Traphagen's Honey
Route 23A West P.O. Box J
Hunter, N.Y. 12442   518-263-4150

PURE . NATURAL . HONEY

NET WT. 2 LBS.

Chapter 3

Honey and Beauty

For centuries, honey had been used by cultures around the world to preserve and enhance natural beauty. During her rule as Queen of Egypt (69 BC-30 BC), Cleopatra indulged in milk and honey baths to keep her skin soft and youthful. In 17th century England, Queen Anne used honey and oil to keep her long hair thick and shiny. As it turns out, recent research has revealed that there is scientific basis for honey's efficacy as a beauty treatment and good reason why these honey concoctions helped preserve these women's legendary beauty.

Today, manufacturers use honey in everything from facial products like moisturizers to products for the body such as soap, bubble bath, and lotions. Not only is honey a widely available, all-natural ingredient, but it's as effective as any manufactured beauty product, too.

Honey is such an effective moisturizer because it is a humectant product which attracts and traps moisture. This makes honey an ideal addition to products that nourish the skin and hair with moisture, such as shampoos, conditioners, cleansers, and creams. Honey also acts as an anti-irritant, helping to calm sensitive skin. It is also gentle enough for baby care products.

When Alexander the Great died, he was returned to Greece in a coffin filled with honey.

But you don't have to be a Queen or spend a fortune to pamper yourself and enjoy the benefits of honey. Try these simple, affordable recipes at home. You'll be feeling like royalty in no time.

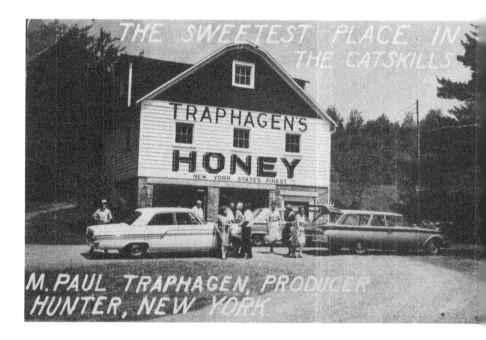

Recipes for Beauty

The following beauty recipes have been created by Christopher Watt, a licensed aesthetician who cares for some of Hollywood's most famous faces, including Halle Berry and Jennifer Lopez. For more of his recipes, visit the National Honey Board website at *www.honey.com.*

For the Face

Green Honey Glow Mask

Makes 2 treatments

Benefits: Beautiful glowing skin that feels youthful and firm.

ingredients

4 cups fresh spinach
1 cup fresh mint
3 Tbsp. honey
1 piece (1-inch) ginger
1 ripe banana
2 egg whites

directions

Rinse spinach thoroughly in colander. Cut and peel ginger, set aside. In food processor or blender combine spinach, mint and ginger. Blend on low setting. Add honey and banana and blend until liquid consistency. Add egg whites and blend until all ingredients are mixed thoroughly. Transfer to porcelain bowl or glass dish. On clean skin apply a small amount of Green Honey Glow to entire face and neck using a fan brush or finger tips. Allow to remain on skin for 15-20 minutes. Rinse and apply appropriate moisturizer. Store covered in refrigerator for up to one week.

"Royal jelly", which is found in many beauty products on the market today, is actually a "food" created by bees to feed tiny baby bees who are destined to become queen bees.

Cucumber Honey Eye Nourisher

Makes 4 treatments

ingredients

1 Tbsp. aloe vera gel
2 tsp. cucumber, peeled with seeds removed
1/2 tsp. chamomile tea
1/2 tsp. honey

directions

Steep chamomile tea in boiling water. Set aside to cool. In food processor or blender combine cucumber, aloe vera and honey. Blend on low setting. Add chamomile tea. Blend until smooth. Apply gently under eyes using ring finger. Store in glass dish covered with plastic wrap in refrigerator for up to one week. Best applied chilled.

Benefits: Reduces puffiness, cools and refreshes contours under eyes.

For the Body
Golden Honey Body Polish

Benefits: Helps to exfoliate and hydrate skin.

ingredients
1/2 cup pure honey
1/2 cup Dead Sea salts (can substitute Epsom salt)*
2/3 cup grapeseed oil (can be found online or at health food stores)

directions
Combine honey, sea salts and grapeseed oil. If you want, crush 2-3 sheets of 24 kt gold leaf until almost powder consistency, add to honey mixture, combine. Apply in bathtub or shower to damp skin. Be sure to work in on rough areas such as elbows, knees and the soles of the feet. Rinse with warm water. Towel dry and apply your favorite moisturizer.

Epsom salt is available online or at health food stores.

Note: **You may add the crushed gold leaf to your favorite moisturizer to further enhance gold's benefits.**

Foaming Vanilla Honey Bath

Makes 4 treatments

Banish the winter blahs and dissolve away the harshness of the day by relaxing in a soothing bath. Honey is nature's silky moisturizer and guaranteed to sweeten your mood!

ingredients

1 cup sweet almond oil, light olive or
sesame oil may be substituted
1/2 cup honey
1/2 cup liquid soap
1 Tbsp. vanilla extract

directions

Measure the oil into a medium bowl, then carefully stir in remaining ingredients until mixture is fully blended. Pour into a clean plastic bottle with a tight-fitting stopper or lid. Shake gently before using. Swirl desired amount into the bathtub under running water—then step in and descend into a warm, silky escape.

> **Honey is a relaxing in a soothing bath.**

Peppermint Honey Feet Treat

Makes 2 treatments

Makes 1 application

Benefits: Aids in circulation of overworked feet. Moisturizes and softens while it soothes and restores tired aching feet.

ingredients

4 Tbsp. aloe vera gel
4 tsp. grated beeswax
2 tsp. honey
2 tsp. fresh mint , optional
6 drops peppermint essential oil
2 drops arnica oil
2 drops camphor oil
2 drops eucalyptus oil

directions

Rinse mint leaves and place on a paper towel to dry. Grind mint using coffee grinder (or by hand using mortar and pestle). Set aside. Melt beeswax using a small double boiler. In a microwave safe glass bowl combine aloe vera and honey, mix well. Stir in beeswax. Let cool. Add mint and oils, stirring until completely mixed. Apply after bath or shower to entire feet and toes. Store remaining feet treat in covered in cool place away from sun or heat. Swirl desired amount into the bathtub under running water—then step in and descend into a warm, silky escape.

For the Hair

Rosemary Honey Hair Conditioner

ingredients

1/2 cup honey
1/4 cup warmed olive oil ,
2 Tbsp. for normal to oily hair
4 drops essential oil of rosemary
1 tsp. xanthum gum (available in health food stores)

directions

Place all the ingredients in a small bowl and mix thoroughly. Pour into a clean plastic bottle with a tight fitting stopper or lid. Apply a small amount at a time to slightly dampened hair. Massage scalp and work mixture through hair until completely coated. Cover hair with a warm towel (towel can be heated in a microwave or dryer) or shower cap; leave on to nourish and condition for 30 minutes. Remove towel or shower cap; shampoo lightly and rinse with cool water. Dry as normal and enjoy shinier, softer and healthier hair the natural way.

The extremes of heat and cold we endure throughout winter can make even the greatest hair look and feel like straw. This nourishing conditioner blends honey for shine, olive oil for moisture and essential oil of rosemary to stimulate hair growth.

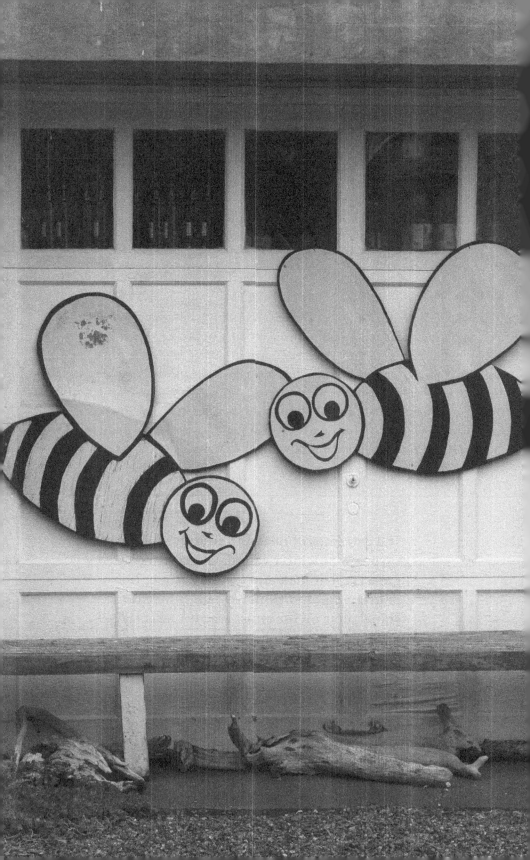

The Recipes

Recipes compliments of The National Honey Board. For nutrition information as well as more delicious recipes, visit their website at *www.honey.com*.

Note: Honey should not be fed to infants under one year of age. Honey is a safe and wholesome food for children and adults.

All of the recipes below were developed for honey, so all you need to do is select a honey and start cooking! The chart below will help you match types of honey to the meal you have in mind.

Light Honey	Flavor Characteristics	Suggested Uses
Alfalfa	Mild flavor; beeswax aroma	Perfect in desserts such as tarts and cookies
Basswood	Green ripening fruit taste; lingering flavor	Whip into butter for a sweet topping
Clove	Sweet flowery flavor and other beverages	Sweeten fresh brewed tea
Fireweed	Delicate and sweet with subtle tea-like notes	Heat slightly, pour onto pancakes or French Toast
Sage	Sweet, clover-like flavor; elegant floral aftertaste	Drizzle on cheese and crackers
Sourwood	Sweet, spicy anise aroma	Stir into fresh fruit salad

Medium Honey	Flavor Characteristics	Suggested Uses
Blueberry	Flowery perfume; lemon aroma and fruity flavor	Slather on warm scones
Brazilian Pepper	Spicy bite	Stir into a fruity salsa
Dandelion	Strong floral flavor	Pour small amounts over vanilla ice cream
Loosestrife	Delicate, sweet flavor over cooked vegetables such as asparagus or carrots	Melt with butter and drizzle
Orange Blossom	Slight citrus taste; delicate waxy aroma	Add to frosty smoothies
Tupelo	Smooth with a complex flora, herbal fruity flavor and aftertaste	Spread onto warm, flaky biscuits

Dark Honey	Flavor Characteristics	Suggested Uses
Avocado	Rich caramelized, flowerly flavor squash soup	Drizzle atop warm butternut
Buckwheat	Pungent, molasses-like flavor; dark and malty	Add into rich barbecue sauces
Eucalyptus	Mildly sweet; with slight menthol flavor	Lightly coast tender lamb shanks
Gallberry	Mild tang	Makes the ideal glaze for fish such as salmon
Wildflower	Floral, pungent flower	Blend into dressing and marinades

Chart courtesy of The National Honey Board website

If you find that you enjoy honey's flavor in meals and want to experiment with substituting honey in recipes that were formulated for sugar, keep the following guidelines in mind.

❀ for best results, use recipes specifically for honey

❀ when substituting honey for sugar, begin by using pure honey for up to half of the granulated sugar called for in the recipe. As you gradually become familiar with using honey instead of sugar, you can eventually replace all the sugar with honey for some recipes. However, you will probably want to progress slowly since honey's high fructose content makes it tastes so much sweet than sugar, meaning you can use less honey than sugar to achieve the same level of sweetness.

❀ cook at an oven temperature 25 degrees lower than the recipe calls for, to prevent over-browning.

❀ to accommodate for honey's liquid quality, reduce any liquid called for in the recipe by 1/4 cup.

❀ for each cup of honey used, add ½ teaspoon baking soda

❀ when measuring honey, coat the measuring cup or measuring spoon with vegetable oil or non-stick spray so that honey will slide out easily without sticking.

Breakfast

Applesauce Breakfast Parfait

Created by Tree Top, Inc.

Makes 2 servings

ingredients

1/2 cup favorite flavored yogurt
3/4 cup granola or other favorite cereal
1/2 cup Tree Top applesauce

directions

In parfait glass layer 2 Tablespoons yogurt, 2 Tablespoons cereal, 2 Tablespoons applesauce; repeat layers. Repeat layering to make second serving.

Colusa Corn Muffins Made with Yogurt

Makes 12 muffins

ingredients

3/4 cup plain yogurt
1/3 cup butter or margarine, melted
1/2 cup honey
2 eggs
3/4 cup all-purpose flour
3/4 cup whole wheat flour
3/4 cup cornmeal
2-1/2 teaspoons baking powder
1/2 teaspoon salt
/2 teaspoon baking soda

directions

Beat together yogurt, butter, honey and eggs in small bowl. Set aside. Combine flours, cornmeal, baking powder, salt and baking soda in large bowl. Add honey mixture. Stir just enough to barely moisten flour. Do not over mix. Spoon batter into paper-lined or greased muffin cups.

Bake in preheated 350°F oven for 20 to 25 minutes or until wooden toothpick inserted near center comes out clean. Remove from pan; cool slightly on wire racks. Serve warm.

Crunchy Honey-Yogurt Breakfast Parfait

Makes 2 servings

ingredients

1 large banana, sliced, divided
1/3 cup honey, divided
1/2 cup plain yogurt, divided
1/2 cup crunchy granola, divided

directions

Reserve several slices of banana for garnish. Layer 1 Tablespoon honey, 1/4 of the pre-sliced banana, 2 Tablespoons yogurt, 2 Tablespoons granola, 1/4 of the sliced banana, 2 Tablespoons yogurt, 1 Tablespoon honey and 2 Tablespoons granola in parfait glass. Repeat for second parfait. Garnish with reserved banana and honey.

Currant Scones

Makes 8 scones

ingredients

2 cups all-purpose flour
1/4 teaspoon baking soda
6 Tablespoons butter, cut into pieces
1/4 cup honey
1 egg plus 1 egg yolk
1 egg white
2 teaspoons baking powder
1/4 teaspoon salt
1 cup currants
1/4 cup nonfat plain yogurt
1/2 teaspoon vanilla or almond extract
Prepared cinnamon-sugar

directions

In large bowl, combine flour, baking powder, baking soda and salt; mix well. Cut in butter until mixture resembles coarse crumbs. Stir in currants. In small bowl, whisk together honey, yogurt, egg, egg yolk and vanilla; add to flour mixture, stirring until just combined. Turn dough onto lightly floured surface; shape into 8-inch circle (approx. 1 inch thick). Cut into 8 wedges. Place on greased baking sheet, at least 1 inch apart. Brush with egg white; sprinkle with cinnamon-sugar.

Bake at 375°F for 15 to 20 minutes or until golden brown.

Honey Granola

Makes 8 cups

ingredients

4 cups old-fashioned rolled oats
2 cups coarsely chopped nuts
1 cup golden raisins
3/4 cup honey
1/2 cup butter or margarine, melted
2 teaspoons ground cinnamon
1 teaspoon vanilla
Salt

directions

Combine oats, nuts and raisins in large mixing bowl; mix well and set aside. Combine honey, butter, cinnamon, vanilla and salt in saucepan; bring to boil and cook one minute. Pour honey mixture over oat mixture and toss until well blended. Spread in lightly greased cookie sheet. Bake at 350°F 20 minutes or until lightly browned; stir every 5 minutes. Cool. Crumble and store in airtight container up to 2 weeks.

Honey Mint Yogurt

ingredients

1 pint plain yogurt
1/4 cup honey
1/2 to 3/4 teaspoons dried mint*, crushed

directions

Combine all ingredients and blend well.

One Tablespoon fresh chopped mint can be substituted.

Honey-Pecan Bran Muffins

Recipe by: Groeb Farms Michigan/The National Honey Board

Makes 12 muffins

ingredients

1 cup fiber cereal, crushed
1 cup milk
1/4 cup vegetable oil
1 egg
1-1/4 cups flour
1/4 cup sugar
1/4 cup honey
1/2 cup pecans, chopped
2 teaspoons baking powder
1/2 teaspoon salt

direction

Heat oven to 400°F. Grease bottom only of 12 medium muffin cups or line with paper cups. Combine cereal and milk. Let stand 5 minutes. Beat in oil and egg. Stir in remaining ingredients just until moistened. Divide batter among muffin cups. Bake until lightly brown, 20 to 30 minutes. Immediately remove from pan to cool.

Spiced Whole Wheat Pancakes

Makes 4 servings

ingredients

3 eggs
2 cups milk
1/4 cup vegetable oil
1/4 cup honey
2-1/2 cups whole wheat flour
5 teaspoons baking powder
1 teaspoon ginger
1 teaspoon cinnamon
1 teaspoon nutmeg
1/4 teaspoon salt

directions

Beat eggs until thick and foamy. Add milk, oil and honey. Beat until
well mixed. Combine flour with remaining ingredients and stir into egg
mixture. Mix well. On greased hot griddle, pour out batter into rounds of
desired size. When batter begins to bubble, turn and cook on other side.
Makes 12 large or 24-30 small pancakes.

Nutty Honey-Bear Wraps

Makes 4 servings

ingredients

1/4 cup honey, plus more to drizzle
1 package (3 oz.) cream cheese, softened
1/4 teaspoon vanilla extract
2 medium bananas
1/3 cup peanut butter chips
4 purchased, ready to use 9-inch crepes or thin pancakes
1/4 cup honey-roasted peanuts, coarsely chopped

directions

In medium bowl, mix honey, cream cheese and vanilla together until well blended. Cut each banana into 1/2-inch thick slices. Gently stir banana slices and peanut butter chips into honey mixture. Lay crepes or pancakes browned side down on a flat work surface. Spoon about 1/2 cup honey-banana filling in a line down one end of each pancake. For each pancake, fold in sides to enclose filling. Place each wrap seam side down on a serving plate. Drizzle each wrap with honey and sprinkle with peanuts. Serve right away.

Strawberry Crepes with Honey Suzette Sauce

Makes 6 servings

ingredients

1/2 cup honey
1/2 cup orange juice
1 Tablespoon lemon juice
2 teaspoons grated orange peel
1-1/2 teaspoons grated lemon peel
1-1/2 teaspoons cornstarch
1 Tablespoon butter or margarine
6 Low-Fat Honey Crêpes
1 pint lemon sorbet or low-fat lemon yogurt
1-1/2 cups fresh strawberries, sliced

directions

In a small saucepan, whisk together honey, orange juice, lemon juice, orange peel, lemon peel and cornstarch until well blended and cornstarch is dissolved. Bring mixture to a boil over medium-high heat, whisking occasionally; cook until mixture thickens. Remove from heat. Whisk in butter or margarine. Cool to room temperature or refrigerate until ready to use.

To assemble, press 1 crepe into each of 6 ramekins or bowls to form a cup. Fill each with 1 scoop of sorbet. Top each with 1/4 cup sliced strawberries and 2 to 3 Tablespoons Honey Suzette Sauce.

Low-Fat Honey Crepes

Makes 6 servings

ingredients

2 cups nonfat milk
1 cup all-purpose flour
2 egg whites
1 egg
1 Tablespoon honey
1 Tablespoon vegetable oil
1/8 teaspoon salt

directions

Combine all ingredients in blender or food processor; blend until smooth. Rub 8-inch nonstick skillet with oiled paper towel or spray lightly with nonstick cooking spray; heat over medium-high heat. Spoon 3 to 4 tablespoons of crepe batter into skillet, tilting and rotating skillet to cover evenly with batter. Cook until edges begin to brown. Turn crepe over and cook until lightly browned. Remove crepe to plate to cool. Repeat process with remaining batter.

Crepes may be refrigerated 3 days or frozen up to 1 month in airtight container.

Appetizers

Honey-Glazed Red Pepper with Goat Cheese

Makes 2 servings

ingredients

1 large sweet red pepper, cored and seeded
1/4 cup thinly sliced onion
2 cloves garlic, crushed
1 Tablespoon olive oil
3 Tablespoons honey
3 Tablespoons red wine vinegar
2 teaspoons dried basil, crushed
1/2 teaspoon salt
pepper to taste
2 whole lettuce leaves
2 oz. goat cheese
Toasted baguettes

directions

Thinly slice red pepper. Sauté pepper, onion and garlic in oil 10 minutes or until onion and pepper are tender. Add honey, vinegar, basil, salt and pepper; cook and stir over medium-high heat until glazed. Serve on lettuce line plates with goat cheese and toasted baguettes.

Honey and Nut Glazed Brie

Makes 16 to 20 servings

ingredients

1/4 cup honey
1 Tablespoon brandy
1/4 cup coarsely chopped pecans
1/4 oz. (about 5-inch diameter) Brie cheese

directions

In a small bowl, combine honey, pecans and brandy. Place cheese on a large ovenproof platter or 9-inch pie plate. Bake in preheated 500°F oven 4 to 5 minutes or until cheese softens. Drizzle honey mixture over top of cheese. Bake 2 to 3 minutes longer or until topping is thoroughly heated. Do not melt cheese.

Serving Suggestions:

Serve with crackers, tart apple wedges and seedless grapes.

Honey Cream Cheese Tea Sandwiches

Makes 7 servings

ingredients

Any variety bread slices
3 oz. cream cheese, softened
2 Tablespoons honey
1/2 teaspoon grated orange peel
Watercress sprigs
Orange peel*, finely julienned

directions

Remove crust from bread; cut into desired shapes. Combine cream cheese, honey and grated orange peel; blend until smooth. Spread cheese mixture on bread; garnish with watercress sprigs and orange peel.

Remove white part of peel.

Golden Nugget Dip

Makes 1 cup

ingredients

1/2 cup honey
1/2 cup spicy brown mustard, prepared

directions

Combine honey and mustard; mix well.

Serving Suggestions:

Serve as a dip for chicken nuggets, vegetables or pretzels.

Bees in the Herb Garden Dip or Dressing

Makes 20 (2 Tablespoon) servings

ingredients

1 pint sour cream
6 Tablespoons honey
2 Tablespoons orange juice, thawed, undiluted
2 Tablespoons Dijon mustard
2 teaspoons cream-style horseradish
2 teaspoons rosemary, crushed
1 teaspoon chervil, crushed
1 teaspoon basil, crushed
3/4 teaspoon salt
1/2 teaspoon white pepper
1/4 teaspoon garlic powder

directions

Combine all ingredients; mix well. Refrigerate, covered, several hours to blend flavors. Stir before using.

Serving Suggestions:

Use as a dip for chips, shrimp, ham cubes, vegetable dippers, ripe olives and pineapple chunks. Use as a salad dressing for green and fruit salads.

Creamy Honey Sesame Dip for Vegetables

Makes 1-1/3 cups

ingredients

3/4 cup nonfat mayonnaise
1/4 cup rice vinegar
1/4 cup honey
3 Tablespoons toasted sesame seeds
1 Tablespoon grated fresh ginger root
1 small garlic, minced
3/4 teaspoon oriental sesame oil
1/8 teaspoon crushed red pepper flakes
Salt, to taste

directions

Whisk together mayonnaise, vinegar and honey in small bowl. Add remaining ingredients; mix thoroughly. Dip may be stored tightly covered in refrigerator up to 1 week.

Serving Suggestions:

Serve with assorted fresh vegetables.

Moroccan Spiced Hummus

Makes 2-1/2 cups

ingredients

2 cans (15 1/2 oz.) garbanzo beans, drained and rinsed
1/3 cup honey
1/4 cup lemon juice
1 teaspoon ground cumin
1 teaspoon minced garlic
1/2 teaspoon salt
2 to 3 Tablespoons fresh cilantro or parsley, chopped
Cayenne pepper
Toasted Pita Triangles or crackers

directions

Combine all ingredients except cilantro and Pita Triangles in a food processor or blender. Process until smooth. Remove mixture to a serving bowl. Stir in chopped cilantro or parsley. Serve with Pita Triangles or crackers.

To Make Pita Triangles: Separate and cut rounds of pita bread to form 2 circles each. Cut each circle into 6 or 8 triangles. Place on a baking sheet. Bake at 400°F about 5 minutes until crisp and lightly browned at edges.

Northwest Bruschetta

Makes 32 slices

ingredients

4 Fuji apples
2 teaspoons vegetable oil
1/4 cup balsamic vinegar
1/2 cup honey
32 1/2-inch thick slices baguette (about 2 inches diameter)
Olive-oil flavored cooking spray
16 very thin slices prosciutto ham (about 10 oz.)
Fresh sage, for garnish

directions

Peel and core apples. Cut each apple into 16 wedges. In large nonstick skillet over medium heat, warm oil and sauté apples 3 minutes or until crisp tender. Add vinegar and cook 3 minutes or until most of the vinegar is evaporated. Add honey and increase heat to high. When honey bubbles, stir gently for 1 minute until apples are soft. Allow apples to cool in honey syrup. With a slotted spoon remove apples; discard syrup.

Heat oven to 400°F. Arrange bread slices on wire rack over cookie sheet. Spray both sides of bread with cooking spray; bake 6 minutes or until edges of bread are golden brown. Remove and arrange on serving platter. Immediately before serving, cut each prosciutto slice into 2- x 1-inch strips. Place one slice of prosciutto on each toast; top with two apple slices. Garnish with fresh sage.

Pear Cheese Tarts with Honey and Hazelnuts

Makes 18 tarts

ingredients

1 box (17.3 oz.) frozen puff pastry
1 pear, cored and quartered
1 lemon, zested and juiced
1/2 cup + 2 Tablespoons Sage honey, divided
8 oz. cream cheese
2 Tablespoons all-purpose flour
2 eggs
1/2 cup chopped hazelnuts
Baking spray

directions

Remove puff pastry from freezer 30 minutes before using. Preheat oven to 400°F.

Cut pear into thin slices. In small bowl, combine pear, 1 Tablespoon lemon juice and 1 Tablespoon honey. Reserve another 1 Tablespoon honey in a small heatproof bowl.

Use a mixer to beat the cream cheese until smooth. Scrape down the sides and add the honey, flour and lemon zest. Mix until smooth. Add the eggs, scrape down the sides again and mix until very smooth.

Cut half of the pastry sheets into 9 squares. Spray a muffin tin with baking spray. Carefully fit 1 square into each muffin cup. Fill each cup with 2 Tablespoons cheese mixture. Cut pear slices to fit muffin tin. Fan 3 or 4 slices of pear over each cup and sprinkle with 1 teaspoon hazelnuts. Freeze 10 to 15 minutes to firm pastry.

Bake cold tarts until pastry is lightly browned and cheese is puffed, about 20 minutes. Cut 9 more pastry squares and repeat filling and baking. Microwave reserved honey 5 seconds on high and drizzle tarts with warm honey.

Let tarts sit 10 to 15 minutes before serving or refrigerate and reheat in a 350°F oven for 10 minutes.

Spicy Honey Drummettes

Makes 7 servings

ingredients

3 lbs. chicken drumettes
1 cup honey
2 Tablespoons curry powder
1 teaspoon ground ginger
1/2 teaspoon cayenne pepper, or to taste

directions

Rinse drummettes and pat dry. Arrange in single layer on a baking
sheet. Bake at 400°F 10 minutes. Meanwhile, in a small bowl, combine
remaining ingredients until well blended. Spoon half of honey mixture
over drummettes; bake 10 minutes. Using tongs, turn drummettes over.
Spoon remaining honey mixture over drummettes; bake 10 minutes
longer. Let cool slightly before serving.

Tortilla Crisps with Honey Dip

Makes 6 servings

ingredients

1/2 cup honey
2 Tablespoons butter or margarine
1 small cinnamon stick
1 piece (1-1/2 x 1/2-inch) orange peel
6 (6-inch) flour tortillas
Vegetable oil

Directions

Combine honey, butter, cinnamon stick and orange peel. Cook over low heat at least 10 minutes. Remove cinnamon stick and peel before serving. Cut each tortilla into six wedges. Deep-fry tortillas, smooth-side up, at 375°F about 30 seconds. Turn and deep-fry 30 seconds longer or until golden brown. Tortillas should puff as soon as they are put in hot oil. Remove from oil to paper towel-lined tray. Serve crisp tortilla with honey dip or spoon dip over chips.

Oven Method: Brush both sides of whole tortillas with vegetable oil. Cut into wedges before baking, if desired. Place on baking sheet and bake at 325°F about 12 minutes or until crisp and browned but not hard.

Main Dishes

Almond Chicken with Honey Lime Sauce

Makes 4 servings

ingredients

2 whole boneless, skinless chicken breasts, halved
2 Tablespoons flour
1 egg
2 teaspoons soy sauce
1/2 teaspoon black pepper
3/4 cup finely ground almonds
3/4 cup corn flake crumbs, crushed
1 Tablespoon vegetable oil
1/2 cup apple juice
juice of 1 lime
2 teaspoons cornstarch
1/4 cup honey

directions

Place chicken breasts between two sheets of plastic wrap or waxed paper. Flatten chicken to 1/2 inch thickness. Dip chicken in flour and shake off excess. Set aside. Combine the egg, soy sauce and pepper in a shallow dish; set aside. In another shallow dish combine ground almonds and corn flake crumbs. Dip chicken in egg mixture to coat and in almond mixture, pressing so the coating adheres to both sides. Brown chicken on both sides in oil in a non-stick skillet over medium-high heat, until chicken is no longer pink and juices run clear when cut with a knife. Remove chicken; set aside. Combine apple juice, lime juice and cornstarch. Add mixture to skillet. Add honey. Cook and stir until thickened and bubbly. Serve chicken with sauce.

Apricot Glazed Chicken

1 (4 to 5 lb.) roasting chicken
1 cup seedless red or green grapes
4 Tablespoons honey
1 can (16 oz.) apricot halves in syrup
1/4 cup butter or margarine, melted
2 teaspoons seasoned salt
1/4 teaspoon black pepper
1/2 cup dry white wine

directions

Rinse chicken in cold water and pat dry with paper towels. Stuff body cavity with 1 cup grapes that have been tossed with 2 Tablespoons honey. Tie legs close to body and fold wing tips back or secure with skewers or twine. Place chicken breast side up on rack in shallow roasting pan.

Drain apricot halves, reserving syrup. Set aside 6 halves for garnish. Process remaining apricots in blender with melted butter, seasoned salt and pepper and remaining 2 Tablespoons honey. Brush over chicken. Pour wine and 1/4 cup apricot syrup in bottom of pan. Cover chicken loosely with tent of aluminum foil. Roast at 350°F for 1-3/4 to 2 hours or until chicken is tender. Baste occasionally with pan drippings to glaze. Remove foil during last 30 minutes of roasting. Serve chicken on platter garnished with clusters of green grapes and apricot halves.

Caribbean Turkey Burgers with Honey Pineapple Chutney

4 servings

Ingredients

1 ripe fresh pineapple, peeled and cut into 1/2" thick slices
1 large onion, peeled and cut into 1/2" slices
2 Tablespoons vegetable oil, divided
1/3 cup honey
1/4 cup red wine vinegar
1 Tablespoon grated orange peel
1 Tablespoon grated fresh ginger
1/4 teaspoon allspice
1/4 cup red bell pepper, minced
1 package (20 oz.) ground turkey
1-1/2 teaspoon Jamaican jerk seasoning
4 Hawaiian sweet sandwich rolls, toasted
Butter lettuce leaves

Directions

To prepare the honey pineapple chutney, begin by brushing pineapple and onion slices with 1-1/2 Tablespoons oil. Grill for about 5 minutes per side over medium-high heat or until lightly charred; remove and let cool slightly. Discard tough pineapple. Finely chop pineapple and onion and place in a medium saucepan with honey, vinegar, orange peel, ginger and allspice; stir well. Bring to a boil; cover and reduce heat and simmer for 45 minutes. Add bell pepper and cook for 10 minutes more; let cool.

In a medium bowl, stir together the ground turkey, 1/2 cup honey pineapple chutney, jerk seasoning and pepper. Shape into 4 large flat patties and brush with remaining oil. Grill over medium coals for 5 to 8 minutes per side or until cooked through. Serve on toasted buns topped with lettuce leaves and a spoonful of chutney.

Easy Homestyle Chicken

Makes 4 servings

ingredients

4 (3-1/2 to 4 oz. each) boneless, skinless chicken breasts
1/2 cup honey
1/2 cup buttermilk baking mix
2 teaspoons ground ginger
1 teaspoon seasoned salt
1/4 teaspoon pepper
2 Tablespoons vegetable oil

directions

Coat chicken with honey; set aside. Combine baking mix, ginger, seasoned salt and pepper; mix well. Roll honey-coated chicken in seasoned mixture. Brown chicken in hot oil in nonstick skillet. Drain excess oil. Place chicken on rack in baking pan and bake at 350°F 20 to 30 minutes or until juices run clear.

Herbed Turkey Breast

Makes 6 servings

ingredients

1/2 cup honey
1/4 cup orange juice
2 Tablespoons butter or margarine, melted
1-1/2 teaspoons sage, dried
1 teaspoon thyme, dried
1 clove garlic, minced
3/4 teaspoon salt
1/4 teaspoon pepper
1 boneless, skinless turkey breast, about 2 lbs.

directions

Preheat broiler. Position oven rack 6 inches from heat source. Combine honey, orange juice, butter, sage, thyme, garlic, salt and pepper. Place turkey breast on rack set in broiler pan. Brush with some of honey mixture. Broil, brushing frequently with remaining mixture, turning turkey once, until no longer pink inside, about 40 minutes. Let stand 5 minutes before slicing.

Honey-Hot Buffalo-Chicken Pizza

Makes 6 servings

ingredients

3/4 cup + 2 Tablespoons prepared tomato-based pizza sauce
1/4 cup honey
1/2 teaspoon hot pepper sauce, or to taste
1 cup diced or shredded, cooked chicken breast
1 tube (10 oz.) refrigerated pizza dough
1 Tablespoon olive oil
3 oz. blue cheese, finely crumbled (3/4 cup)
1/2 cup finely diced celery

directions

Heat pizza sauce and honey; remove from heat. Stir in hot pepper sauce.
Mix 2 Tablespoons sauce with chicken; reserve. Shape pizza dough
according to package directions for thin-crusted pizza. Brush pizza shell
with 1 Tablespoon olive oil. Spread remaining 3/4 cup sauce over dough.
Scatter reserved chicken over sauce. Bake at 500°F until lightly browned,
about 10 minutes. Remove from oven. Sprinkle pizza with cheese, then
celery. Cut pizza into 6 wedges.

Low-Fat Chicken and Asparagus Crepes

Makes 6 servings

ingredients

1 cup nonfat sour cream
6 Tablespoons honey
1 Tablespoon lemon juice
2 teaspoons curry powder
1/2 teaspoon salt
1/8 teaspoon ground red pepper, or to taste
1-1/2 lbs. boneless, skinless chicken breasts, cooked
 and cut into 1-inch cubes
1 lb. asparagus, cooked, cooled and cut into 1-inch pieces
1 red bell pepper, chopped
2 green onions, thinly sliced
Low-Fat Honey Crêpes
Fresh parsley or cilantro, optional

directions

Combine sour cream, honey, lemon juice, curry powder, salt and ground red pepper in large bowl until well blended. Add chicken, asparagus, bell pepper and green onions; toss to coat evenly with dressing. Spoon 1/3 cup chicken mixture down center of each crepe. Fold and roll crepes to enclose chicken mixture. Garnish with parsley sprigs, if desired.

Slam Dunk'n Chicken Strips

Makes 6 servings

ingredients

1/4 cup honey
1/4 cup teriyaki sauce
1-1/2 cups plain dry bread crumbs
1 lb. boneless chicken breasts, cut into 1-inch strips
Salt and pepper
Nonstick cooking spray

directions

Preheat oven to 425°F. Lightly spray a baking sheet with cooking spray. In shallow bowl, whisk together honey and teriyaki sauce. Pour bread crumbs into separate bowl. Set bowls aside. Season chicken strips with salt and pepper as desired. Dip strips in honey mixture, then in bread crumbs. Arrange chicken strips on baking sheet; lightly coat with cooking spray. Bake 12 to 15 minutes or until cooked through. Serve with a favorite dipping sauce.

Teriyaki-Glazed Turkey Burgers

Makes 4 servings

ingredients

1/3 cup honey
1/4 cup soy sauce
1-1/2 teaspoons grated fresh ginger root
1 teaspoon minced garlic
1 lb. ground turkey
1/2 cup finely chopped celery
1/4 cup thinly sliced green onion
4 hamburger buns, toasted

directions

In a small bowl, combine honey, soy sauce, ginger, and garlic until well blended. In a separate bowl, mix together turkey, celery, and green onions. Blend in 3 Tablespoons honey glaze mixture. Divide mixture into 4 patties, 1/2- to 3/4-inch thick. Place patties on a well-oiled grill, 4-6 inches from hot coals. Grill, turning 2 to 3 times, brushing generously with glaze, until patties are well browned and cooked through. Serve on toasted buns.

A Honey of a Chili

Makes 8 servings

ingredients

1 package (15 oz.) firm tofu
1 Tablespoon vegetable oil
1 cup chopped onion
3/4 cup chopped green bell pepper
2 cloves garlic, finely chopped
2 Tablespoons chili powder
1 teaspoon ground cumin
1 teaspoon salt
1/2 teaspoon dried oregano
1/2 teaspoon crushed red pepper flakes
1 can (28 oz.) diced tomatoes, undrained
1 can (15-1/2 oz.) red kidney beans, undrained
1 can (8 oz.) tomato sauce
1/4 cup honey
2 Tablespoons red wine vinegar

directions

Using a cheese grater, shred tofu and freeze in zippered bag or airtight container. Thaw tofu; place in a strainer and press out excess liquid. In large saucepan or dutch oven, heat oil over medium-high heat until hot; cook and stir onion, green pepper and garlic 3 to 5 minutes or until vegetables are tender and begin to brown. Stir in chili powder, cumin, salt, oregano and crushed red pepper. Stir in tofu: cook and stir 1 minute. Stir in diced tomatoes, kidney beans, tomato sauce, honey and vinegar.

Bring to a boil; reduce heat and simmer, uncovered, 15 to 20 minutes, stirring occasionally.

Garden Stir-Fry

Makes 6 to 8 servings

ingredients

1 Tablespoon vegetable oil
1 clove garlic, minced
1 small onion, vertically sliced
3 medium zucchini, julienned
1 medium yellow squash, julienned
1 large carrot, julienned
1/4 cup honey
2 Tablespoons lemon juice
1 teaspoon salt
1 teaspoon pepper

directions

Heat oil in a heavy skillet or stir-fry pan over high heat. Add garlic and onion and cook until fragrant, 1-2 minutes. Add zucchini, yellow squash, and carrot and stir-fry until vegetables are crisp-tender.

Honey-Roasted
Red Pepper Couli

Makes 6 servings -

ingredients

5 red bell peppers, cored, seeded and sliced in half
3 Tablespoons olive oil
2 Tablespoons olive oil, used later in recipe
1 Tablespoon honey
1/3 cup honey, used later in recipe
2 teaspoons balsamic vinegar
1 teaspoon teriyaki sauce
1/2 teaspoon liquid smoke

directions

In mixing bowl, add red peppers to 3 Tablespoons of olive oil and 1
Tablespoon honey. Coat well. Place peppers on a heated grill and cook,
turning several times. Peppers are done when charred on each side and
softened. Remove peppers from grill, place in plastic bag and seal. Set
aside for 15 minutes, then peel and discard the skin from the peppers
and transfer them to a food processor. Add 1/3 cup honey, vinegar,
teriyaki sauce and liquid smoke. Process 30 seconds and, with processor
running, slowly add 2 Tablespoons olive oil in a steady stream. Couli can
be made a day ahead and refrigerated in an airtight container.

Stuffed Sweet Peppers

Makes 4 servings

ingredients

1 Tablespoon vegetable or olive oil
3/4 cup uncooked long-grain rice
4 green onions, thinly sliced
1/4 cup finely chopped fresh parsley
1/4 teaspoon ground cinnamon
1/4 teaspoon black pepper
1/4 teaspoon salt
1 can (14-1/2 oz.) vegetable broth
4 medium green bell peppers, cut lengthwise in half, seeded
1 can (28 oz.) crushed tomatoes in pureé
1/4 cup honey
1/2 teaspoon crushed red pepper flakes
1 can (8-3/4 oz.) garbanzo beans, drained
1/3 cup dried currants or raisins

directions

In large saucepan, heat oil over medium-high heat until hot; cook and stir rice, onion and parsley 3 to 5 minutes, or until rice begins to brown. Stir in cinnamon, pepper and salt. Gradually add vegetable broth. Bring to a boil, reduce heat, cover and simmer for 18 to 20 minutes, or until liquid is absorbed and rice is cooked through.

Meanwhile, cook green pepper halves in boiling water 5 to 7 minutes or until peppers are crisp-tender; drain. Combine tomatoes, honey, and crushed red pepper in 13 x 9-inch baking pan; mix well. Remove 1/4 cup sauce; set aside. Arrange pepper halves on sauce in baking pan.

When rice is cooked, remove from heat; stir in garbanzo beans, dried currants and reserved 1/4 cup sauce. Divide rice evenly among pepper halves in baking pan. Cover pan tightly with foil. Bake at 350°F for 30 minutes.

Thai Noodles with Tofu and Snow Peas

Makes 6 servings

ingredients

1 package (15 oz.) extra firm tofu, drained, pressed and cut into 1/2-inch pieces
1 package (9 oz.) fresh Asian-style noodles
4 oz. snow peas, trimmed and diagonally cut
1/4 cup chopped fresh cilantro

Tips:

1 package (8 oz.) dried fettuccine may be substituted for Asian-style noodles. Prepare according to package directions, adding snow peas during last 2 or 3 minutes of cooking.

Marinade:
1/4 cup honey
2 Tablespoons soy sauce
1 Tablespoon sesame oil
1/2 teaspoon crushed red pepper

1/3 cup rice vinegar
2 Tablespoons peanut butter
2 Tablespoons vegetable oil
2 cloves garlic, finely chopped
1/4 teaspoon ground ginger

directions

In a medium bowl, combine marinade ingredients. Add tofu; marinate 30 minutes.

Cook noodles and snow peas in 3 quarts boiling water 1 to 2 minutes, or until peas are crisp-tender; drain. Rinse with cold water; drain. Place in a large bowl; add tofu and marinade. Toss gentle to coat. Add cilantro; toss to coat.

Vegetables with Spicy Honey Peanut Sauce

Makes 6 servings

ingredients

1/2 cup honey
1/4 cup peanut butter
2 Tablespoons soy sauce
1 Tablespoon chopped fresh cilantro
1/8 teaspoon crushed red pepper flakes
4 cups broccoli florets
4 cups sliced carrots
4 cups snow peas
6 cups cooked white rice

directions

Combine honey, peanut butter, soy sauce, cilantro and red pepper in small bowl; mix well and set aside. Steam vegetables until crisp-tender; drain well. Toss steamed vegetables with peanut sauce in large bowl. Serve immediately over rice.

Beef and Potato Tzimmes

Makes 6 servings

ingredients

2 Tablespoons Vegetable oil, divided
2 lbs. stew meat, cut in 1-1/2-inch chunks
2 cups chopped onion
2 cups sliced (1-inch thick) carrots
2 teaspoons garlic salt
Water
2 cups cubed (1-inch thick) potato
2 cups cubed (1-inch thick) sweet potato
1/3 cup honey
1/2 teaspoon ground cinnamon
1/8 teaspoon ground pepper
4 oz. dried apricots
4 oz. pitted prunes
2 Tablespoons flour, optional
2 Tablespoons chopped parsley

directions

Heat 1 tablespoon of oil in heavy 5-quart pot over medium heat. Add beef and brown on all sides. Remove beef from pan, add remaining oil, if necessary, and sauté onion until tender. Return beef to pan; add carrots, salt and about 4 cups water to cover ingredients. Bring to a boil, reduce heat, cover and simmer 1 hour. Add potatoes, sweet potatoes, honey, cinnamon and pepper; stir and return to a boil. Reduce heat and simmer, partially covered, 30 minutes or until potatoes are barely cooked. Add dried fruit and simmer, uncovered, 30 minutes or until beef is tender. Liquid should be slightly thickened. If necessary, dissolve flour in 3 tablespoons water and stir into stew; return to simmer, stirring frequently. Sprinkle with parsley before serving, if desired.

Honey & Ginger Marinated Flank Steak with Horseradish Sauce

Makes 4 servings

ingredients

1/4 cup soy sauce
1/3 cup honey
2 Tablespoons balsamic vinegar
1-1/2 teaspoons garlic powder, or 1 clove garlic, minced
2 Tablespoons fresh grated ginger
1/2 cup canola oil
2 lbs. flank steak

directions

Combine soy sauce, honey, vinegar, garlic powder, ginger and oil in a container with a tight lid. Shake to mix well. Make light diagonal slashes on each side of the flank steak in a diamond pattern. Place meat in a small pan and pour marinade over it. Cover and place in the refrigerator for at least 4 hours. Prepare the grill for cooking on medium-high heat. Cook the steak about 6 to 8 minutes on each side, remove from grill and let steak rest for 5 minutes. Slice thinly on the diagonal and serve with Sweet Horseradish Sauce.

Sweet Horseradish Sauce

Makes 4 servings

ingredients

1/4 cup honey
1/4 cup mayonnaise
1/2 cup whipped cream
3 Tablespoons prepared horseradish
1 teaspoon Dijon mustard
1/4 teaspoon salt
1 teaspoon balsamic vinegar

directions

In small bowl, mix honey and mayonnaise until smooth, fold in whipped cream. Stir in horseradish, mustard, salt and vinegar. Mix well. Store in refrigerator until ready to use.

Honey-Glazed Lamb and Zucchini Gratin

Makes 8 servings

ingredients

8 kosher lamb chops
4 Tablespoons olive oil, divided
3 cups diced onion
3 cups diced zucchini
2 cups diced fresh tomatoes
4 Tablespoons chopped fresh mint, divided
2/3 cup honey
2 teaspoons ground cumin
1 teaspoon minced garlic
Salt and ground black pepper, to taste

directions

Season lamb chops with salt and pepper. Heat 2 Tablespoons olive oil in a skillet over medium-high heat. Brown chops 5 to 7 minutes on each side; remove from pan and keep warm. Drain fat, leaving any browned bits. Add remaining oil and onion; cook over medium heat until softened. Stir in zucchini and cook until tender-crisp. Stir in tomatoes and 2 Tablespoons mint; cook about 1 minute. Meanwhile, in small saucepan, combine honey, remaining mint, cumin, garlic, 1/4 teaspoon salt, and pepper to taste. Cook over low heat until honey is thinned. To serve, spoon vegetable mixture onto a plate, top with lamb chop and drizzle with honey glaze.

Meatloaf with Pine Nuts

Makes 6 to 8 servings

Ingredients

1/4 cup plus 1 Tablespoon honey
2 lbs. ground chuck or ground round
1 cup finely chopped onion
1/2 cup dry bread crumbs, softened in 1/2 cup milk
2 large eggs
1/3 cup pine nuts
1/2 cup sun dried tomatoes, simmered in boiling water 5 minutes, drained and chopped
1 Tablespoon thyme
1-1/2 teaspoons ground cumin
1-1/2 teaspoons black pepper

directions

Combine 1/4 cup honey with all other ingredients until evenly mixed. Press into 9 x 5-inch metal loaf pan. Drizzle remaining 1 Tablespoon honey over meatloaf and spread to cover top. Bake uncovered at 400°F for 50 to 60 minutes or until meat thermometer inserted into center registers 155 to 160°F. Let rest 5 minutes.

Peppered Asiago Bacon Burgers with Honeyed Arugula

Makes 6 servings

ingredients

2 lbs. ground chuck
1 cup asiago cheese, grated
2 teaspoons Salt, divided
2 teaspoons Freshly ground black pepper
1 Tablespoon Worcestershire sauce
1/3 cup honey
2 Tablespoons lemon juice
6 cups arugula leaves
6 sesame seed buns
1/4 cup mayonnaise
6 slices bacon, cooked, crisp
6 slices tomato

directions

Combine ground chuck, asiago cheese, 1 teaspoon of the salt, pepper and Worcestershire sauce in a large bowl. Form into 6 patties. Grill on closed grill until cooked through (about 4-5 minutes per side).

In a medium bowl, whisk together honey, lemon juice and remaining salt. Add the arugula and toss to coat. Toast the buns lightly on the grill. Divide the mayonnaise between each of the six rolls, spreading on the bottom half of each. Place patties on buns, add one piece of bacon on top of each burger and top each with a slice of tomato. Evenly divide the honeyed arugula between each patty. Place bun tops on and serve.

Pepper-Crusted Sliced Steak on Texas Toast with Honey-Roasted Red Pepper Couli

Makes 6 servings

ingredients

2 lbs. London broil beef, 1-inch thick
1/4 cup melted butter
1/4 cup coarse ground black pepper
Nonstick cooking spray
12 slices Texas toast, grill-toasted per instructions on box

directions

Wash and trim steak. Use a meat mallet or tenderizer to tenderize the steak. Brush 1 side of steak with melted butter. Press black pepper onto same side of beef to form crust. Spray barbecue grill grid with non-stick spray and grill steak on covered grill for 8 to 10 minutes. Turn, using care to avoid scraping off pepper. Grill an additional 18 to 20 minutes on the other side for medium-rare or longer until desired doneness is reached, turning again if necessary. Remove from grill and set beef on cutting board. Rest for 5 minutes, then cut steak across the grain into thin slices. To assemble sandwiches, lay strips of beef, pepper side up, on one slice of Texas toast. Spoon couli over the beef and top with second toast slice.

Tips

Texas toast is available in grocer's frozen baked goods section or make your own with 1-inch thick sliced bread by spreading one side of the bread with garlic butter and toasting bread over the grill.

Broiled Fish with Tangy Sweet 'n Sour Sauce

Makes 8 servings

ingredients

1/2 cup water
1/2 cup honey
1/4 cup lemon juice or rice vinegar
1/4 cup dry white wine
1 Tablespoon cornstarch
1 teaspoon garlic salt
1/2 teaspoon grated lemon peel
1 Tablespoon chopped fresh cilantro, tarragon, thyme or basil
2 lbs. red snapper fillets or cod fillets

directions

Combine all ingredients except cilantro and fish in small saucepan; cook and stir over medium heat until mixture boils and thickens. Simmer 2 minutes. Add cilantro; mix well. Remove sauce from heat and keep warm. Place fish on lightly oiled baking sheet. Broil 4 to 6 inches from heat source 10 minutes per inch of thickness or until fish turns opaque and flakes easily when tested with fork. Spoon sauce over fish to serve.

Easy Salmon Burgers with Honey Barbecue Sauce

Makes 2 servings

ingredients

2 hamburger buns, toasted
1/3 cup honey
1/3 cup ketchup
1-1/2 teaspoons cider vinegar
1 teaspoon prepared horseradish
1/4 teaspoon minced garlic
1/8 teaspoon crushed red pepper flakes, optional
1 can (7-1/2 oz.) salmon, drained
1/2 cup dried bread crumbs
1/4 cup chopped onion
3 Tablespoons chopped green bell pepper
1 egg white

directions

In small bowl, combine honey, ketchup, vinegar, horseradish, garlic and red pepper flakes until well blended. Set aside half of sauce. In separate bowl, mix together salmon, bread crumbs, onion, green pepper and egg white. Blend in 2 tablespoons remaining sauce. Divide salmon mixture into 2 patties, 1/2- to 3/4-inch thick. Place patties on well-oiled grill, 4 to 6 inches from hot coals. Grill, turning 2 to 3 times and basting with sauce, until burgers are browned and cooked through. Or place patties on lightly greased baking sheet. Broil 4 to 6 inches from heat source, turning 2 to 3 times and basting with remaining sauce, until cooked through. Place on hamburger buns and serve with reserved sauce.

Firecracker Shrimp

Makes 4 servings

ingredients

1/3 cup honey
1/4 cup soy sauce
1 Tablespoon rice wine vinegar
2 teaspoons cornstarch
2 teaspoons grated orange peel
1/4 teaspoon crushed red pepper flakes, or to taste
1 Tablespoon vegetable oil
4 cloves garlic, minced
2 teaspoons minced fresh ginger
1 red bell pepper, seeded and chopped
1 cup snow peas, cut into 1-inch pieces
1-1/2 lbs. shrimp, peeled and deveined
3 green onions, cut into 1-inch pieces
6 cups cooked white rice, optional

directions

In small bowl, whisk together honey, soy sauce, vinegar, cornstarch, orange peel and red pepper flakes until thoroughly mixed and cornstarch is dissolved. Set aside. Heat oil in wok or large, heavy skillet over medium-high heat. Stir in garlic and ginger; stir-fry until fragrant, about 1 minute. Add bell pepper and snow peas; stir-fry 1 minute until crisp-tender. Add shrimp and green onions; stir-fry until shrimp just turns pink, about 1 minute. Stir in reserved soy sauce mixture; cook and stir until sauce boils and thickens. Serve over cooked rice, if desired.

Kiwifruit & Pepper Sauté with Whitefish

Makes 4 servings

ingredients

1/2 cup corn flake crumbs
Salt and pepper, to taste
1 lb. whitefish fillet, thawed and cubed
1/4 cup milk
1/4 cup chicken broth or water
3/4 teaspoon cornstarch
1/4 cup diced onion
2 teaspoons vegetable oil
1/2 cup diced yellow or green pepper
1/4 cup thinly sliced carrots
1 Tablespoon packed brown sugar
1-1/2 teaspoons vinegar
2 kiwifruit, pared and sliced

directions

Combine cornflakes crumbs, salt and pepper. Dip fish into milk and coat with crumb mixture. Place on greased baking sheet; bake at 375°F for 10 to 15 minutes or until fish is golden and flakes when tested with a fork. Arrange on serving platter. Combine water and cornstarch; set aside. Sauté onions in oil 1 minute; stir in pepper, carrot, brown sugar and vinegar. Sauté 2 minutes. Stir in cornstarch mixture and cook and stir until thickened; remove from heat. Stir in kiwifruit. Spoon over fish.

Sweet Spicy Salmon with Honeyed Mango Salsa

Makes 4 to 6 servings

ingredients

1 large ripe mango, peeled and chopped
1/4 cup red bell pepper, finely chopped
1/4 cup red onion, finely chopped
2 Tbsp. fresh cilantro, chopped
2 Tbsp. fresh lime juice, divided
1 Tbsp. honey
1 small jalapeno pepper, seeded and minced
1/3 cup honey
2 Tbsp. Mexican hot sauce
4 (4 to 6-oz.) salmon fillets

directions

To prepare the salsa, combine the mango, bell pepper, red onion, cilantro, 1 tablespoon of lime juice, 1 tablespoon honey and jalapeno in a medium bowl. Stir well and refrigerate until ready to use. Whisk together the honey, hot sauce and remaining lime juice in a small bowl. Rinse salmon and pat dry; brush liberally with honey mixture. Place skin side up on a well oiled grill over medium coals; cook for 2 to 3 minutes until lightly charred. Turn and cook for 8 to 10 minutes more, basting liberally with sauce during cooking. Remove from grill and transfer to a serving platter. Top with mango salsa.

Honey Apple Chutney Pork Chops

Makes 4 servings

ingredients

4 pork chops, lean, center-cut, about 1-1/2 lbs
1 Tablespoon vegetable oil
1 cup onion, chopped
3 cloves garlic, minced
1 tart, green apple, cored and diced
3 Tablespoons cider vinegar
1/4 cup honey
1/4 cup currants
Salt and pepper, to taste

directions

In large, heavy skillet, brown pork chops on both sides in oil over medium heat. Remove chops and keep warm. Add onion and garlic to pan. Cook and stir until lightly browned. Add apple. Cook and stir until soft and liquid has evaporated, about 3 minutes. Add vinegar, stirring to dislodge caramelized juiced. Stir in honey and currants; season to taste with salt and pepper. Return pork chops to pan, spooning chutney over chops. Cook until chops are cooked through and glaze is syrupy, about 5 more minutes.

Honey Glazed Ham

Makes 4 servings

ingredients

2 (8 oz. each) ham steaks, cooked
1/4 cup honey
3 Tablespoons water
1-1/2 teaspoons dry mustard
1/2 teaspoon ground ginger
1/4 teaspoon ground cloves

directions

Pan-fry or broil ham steaks until lightly browned and thoroughly heated. Remove ham from skillet or broiler pan. Combine honey, water, spices; add to pan drippings and bring to a boil. Simmer 1 to 2 minutes. Brush over ham and serve with remaining sauce.

Honey Ginger Roasted Pork

Makes 6 servings

ingredients

1/4 cup honey
2 Tablespoons cider vinegar
2 Tablespoons fresh ginger root or ground ginger, grated
2 to 2-1/4 lbs. boneless pork loin roast, whole

directions

Combine honey, vinegar and ginger; mix well. Sprinkle pork with
salt and pepper; brush generously with honey mixture. Bake at 325°F
about 1 hour or to 170 degrees internal temperature. Brush with honey
mixture every 15 minutes. Let stand 10 minutes before slicing.

Mediterranean Wrap

Makes 4 servings

ingredients

1 cup uncooked couscous

1/2 cup raisins

2 cups shredded lettuce

1/4 cup olive oil

2 Tablespoons chopped fresh parsley

1 teaspoon grated lemon peel

4 pita bread pockets, split into 8 rounds

1/2 cup chopped almonds, toasted

3 cups cooked, shredded pork roast

1/4 cup honey

1/4 cup lemon juice

1 teaspoon curry powder

Salt and pepper, to taste

1 cup hummus

directions

Cook couscous according to package directions. In medium bowl, gently combine couscous, almonds, raisins, pork* and lettuce. In small bowl, whisk together honey, olive oil, lemon juice, parsley, curry powder and lemon peel. Season with salt and pepper. Mix 1/4 cup dressing into couscous mixture. To assemble wraps, lay pita rounds split side up on work surface. Spread each with 2 Tablespoons hummus. Spoon approximately 1/2 cup couscous mixture down center of each pita round. Drizzle with 1 Tablespoon dressing and fold in sides to wrap.

*Preparing Pork for Your Favorite Wrap: Season a 1-1/2 lb. boneless pork roast with salt and pepper; brown on all sides in a hot nonstick skillet with a little olive oil. Add 1/2 cup chicken broth or water to pan, lower heat, cover tightly and simmer for 1-1/2 hours, until roast is very tender. Check pan occasionally for liquid level; if broth has evaporated, add a little more to pan to maintain a moist cooking environment. Remove roast from pan, let cool slightly and shred or chop pork coarsely. A 1-1/2 lb. roast will yield 4 cups of pork. Use immediately or cover and refrigerate up to 4 days, until ready to use. Serve cold or reheated.

Serving Suggestions

Optional toppings include yogurt and shredded cucumber.

Pork Tenderloin with Honey-Balsamic Sauce

Makes 6 to 8 servings

ingredients

2 pork tenderloins
1/4 cup paprika
1/4 cup kosher salt
1/4 cup fresh ground pepper
1 Tablespoon garlic powder
1 Tablespoon onion powder
1 teaspoon ground chipotle peppers
1/3 cup seedless raspberry preserves, for sauce
1/3 cup Dijon mustard, for sauce
1/3 cup balsamic vinegar, for sauce
1/3 cup honey

directions

Wash tenderloins and pat dry. Combine dry rub ingredients together then apply half of dry rub to each tenderloin. Set aside and let come to room temperature (about 1 hour).

Prepare grill for direct cooking over medium-high heat.

Cook tenderloins over medium-high heat for 10 minutes. Turn and cook 10 more minutes. Remove from heat and wrap in aluminum foil for 10 minutes.

Combine raspberry preserves, mustard, vinegar and honey in a small saucepan. Heat over medium-high heat until almost boiling, then remove.

To serve, slice tenderloin 1/4 to 1/2-inch thick and fan out on plate. Drizzle warm sauce over slices.

Salads and Dressings

Classic Honey Mustard Dressing

Makes 2-1/2 cups

ingredients

1-1/4 cups fat-free mayonnaise
1/3 cup honey
1 Tablespoon vinegar
2/3 cup vegetable oil
1 teaspoon onion flakes
2 Tablespoons chopped fresh parsley
2 Tablespoons prepared mustard

directions

In small bowl, whisk together all ingredients until blended. Cover and refrigerate until ready to serve.

Honey Balsamic Vinaigrette

Makes 1 cup

ingredients

1/2 cup canned apricots, drained
1/3 cup balsamic vinegar or red wine vinegar
1/4 cup honey
2 teaspoons Dijon mustard
1 clove garlic
1 teaspoon dry Italian seasoning
1/4 teaspoon salt and pepper
1 Tablespoon olive oil

directions

In blender or food processor, combine apricots, vinegar, honey, mustard, garlic and seasonings; blend until smooth. With motor running, slowly drizzle in olive oil until combined.

Honey-Dijon Dressing

Makes 4 servings

ingredients

1/4 cup honey
1/4 cup balsamic vinegar
3 Tablespoons Dijon-style mustard
1 Tablespoon chopped fresh thyme
1 Tablespoon vegetable oil
1/4 teaspoon freshly ground black pepper

directions

Combine all ingredients in a small bowl; mix well. Set aside.

Serving Suggestions
Try with Farmers Market Chicken Salad

Honey Vinaigrette II

Makes 4 servings

ingredients

2 Tablespoons honey
1/2 Tablespoon champagne or white wine vinegar
1 Tablespoon shallot, finely chopped
1/4 teaspoon salt
1/8 teaspoon pepper
3 Tablespoons olive oil

directions

Whisk together honey and next 4 ingredients; whisk in oil.

Farmers Market Chicken Salad

Makes 4 servings

ingredients

Nonstick cooking spray
1-1/2 cups toasted wheat germ
1 teaspoon garlic powder
1 teaspoon salt
1/2 teaspoon freshly ground black pepper
3 egg whites
2 Tablespoons water
1 lb. boneless, skinless chicken breasts, cut into 1-inch wide strips
6 cups mixed salad greens, torn into bite sized pieces
2 cups red or yellow cherry tomatoes, halved

1-1/2 cups thin green beans, snow/sugar snap peas, cucumbers or sliced bell peppers

directions

Heat oven to 400°F. Spray a large baking sheet with cooking spray.

For chicken, combine wheat germ, garlic powder, salt and pepper in a shallow dish; mix well. In another shallow dish, beat egg whites and water until frothy. Dip chicken strips into egg mixture then in wheat germ mixture. Dip and coat chicken again, coating thoroughly; place on baking sheet. Lightly spray with cooking spray. Bake 12 to 15 minutes or until chicken is no longer pink in center.

To assemble salad, arrange greens, tomatoes and green beans on serving platter; top with warm chicken. Drizzle Honey-Dijon Dressing over salad.

Fiesta Salad
with Sherry Vinaigrette

Makes 4 servings

ingredients

1/4 cup honey
1/4 cup sherry vinegar
1/2 teaspoon ground cumin
2 cups chopped romaine lettuce
1 avocado, peeled and sliced
1 cucumber, peeled and sliced
1 bunch radishes, sliced
Salt and ground black pepper, to taste

directions

In small bowl, whisk together honey, vinegar and cumin; set aside. In large bowl, combine lettuce, avocado, cucumber and radishes. Add dressing; toss to coat.

Fruit Salad
with Honey Lime Dressing

Makes 4 servings
Preparation Time: 10 minutes

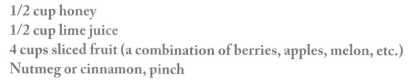

ingredients

1/2 cup honey
1/2 cup lime juice
4 cups sliced fruit (a combination of berries, apples, melon, etc.)
Nutmeg or cinnamon, pinch

directions

In blender or food processor, combine honey, juice and seasoning; blend until smooth. In medium bowl, toss fruit with dressing and chill until ready to serve.

Grilled Portobello Mushroom Salad with Greens, Honey Vinaigrette and Roquefort

Makes 4 servings

ingredients

1/3 cup honey
1/4 cup balsamic vinegar
3 Tablespoons soy sauce
2 cloves garlic, coarsely chopped
1/3 cup olive oil
4 (3 to 4-inch) portobello mushrooms, cleaned with stems removed
1/4 cup bacon, chopped (or 1 ounce cooked bacon bits)
8 cups mixed baby greens
Honey Vinaigrette, recipe follows
1/2 cup crumbled Roquefort or blue cheese
Snipped chives, for garnish

directions

Make marinade: In container of electric blender, blend honey, vinegar, soy sauce, garlic and 1/4 cup oil until smooth; set aside.

Brush mushrooms on both sides with 1-1/2 Tablespoons oil; place on indoor grill or in preheated nonstick skillet over medium-high heat. Cook about 5 minutes, turning occasionally, just until tender. Transfer to non-reactive container, gill sides up. Pour marinade over mushrooms; cover and refrigerate 2 to 4 hours, basting with marinade occasionally. If using raw bacon, sauté bacon until lightly browned. Remove to paper towels to drain; set aside. Drain, then reheat mushrooms 1 to 2 minutes on indoor or outdoor grill, turning once.

In large bowl, toss greens with 1/3 cup (or to taste) Honey Vinaigrette. Divide greens equally among four individual serving plates. Halve mushrooms. Prop one half on the other on each salad. Divide cheese and cooked bacon bits among the salads. Sprinkle with chives.

Honey-Dressed Couscous Salad

Makes 5 to 6 servings

ingredients

1-1/4 cups water
1 cup couscous
2 cups shredded cooked chicken breast (approx. 8 oz.)
1 can (15-1/2 oz.) garbanzo beans, rinsed and drained
2 medium carrots, shredded
3 green onions, thinly sliced
3 Tablespoons finely chopped parsley
1/3 cup fresh lemon juice
1/4 cup honey
2 Tablespoons Olive oil
2 teaspoons freshly grated lemon peel
1 teaspoon salt
1/4 teaspoon ground black pepper

directions

In a small bowl, combine dressing ingredients; mix until blended. Set aside.

In a small saucepan, bring water to a boil. Remove from heat; stir in couscous. Cover and let stand 5 minutes; fluff with fork. Remove to large bowl; let cool. Stir in chicken, garbanzo beans, carrots, onion and parsley. Add dressing; toss to coat.

Mixed Melon Salad

Makes 6 servings

ingredients

6 cups assorted melon balls, such as cantaloupe and honeydew
2/3 cup honey
1/3 cup white wine vinegar with tarragon
1/8 teaspoon ground ginger

directions

In a large bowl, combine dressing ingredients; mix until blended. Add melon balls; toss lightly to coat.

Primavera Pasta Salad

Makes 6 servings

ingredients

1-1/2 Tablespoons olive oil
1-1/2 Tablespoons butter or margarine
1-1/2 cups broccoli florets
2 cloves garlic, minced
2 tomatoes, seeded and diced
3/4 cup julienne zucchini
1/2 cup julienne carrots
1/4 cup honey
1/4 cup lemon juice
1-1/2 teaspoons grated lemon peel
3/4 teaspoon dried basil, crushed
3/4 teaspoon dried oregano, crushed
6 oz. linguine pasta, cooked
Parmesan cheese, grated
Salt and pepper, to taste

directions

Heat oil and butter in a large skillet over medium-high heat; add broccoli and garlic and stir-fry 2 minutes. Reduce heat to low and add tomatoes, zucchini, carrot, honey, lemon juice, lemon peel and seasonings. Simmer about 4 minutes or until vegetables are tender, stirring gently. Toss with noodles; cool. Sprinkle with parmesan cheese. Serve at room temperature or chilled.

Roasted Pepper Salad with Honey-Balsamic Dressing

Makes 4 servings

ingredients

3 red bell peppers, or a combination of red, yellow
and green bell peppers
2 Tablespoons olive oil, divided
1/4 cup golden raisins
1/4 cup balsamic vinegar
2 Tablespoons honey
1/2 teaspoon dried basil
1/2 teaspoon garlic salt
1/4 teaspoon dried oregano

directions

Cut bell peppers lengthwise in half; cut each half lengthwise into 2 or
3 pieces. Arrange peppers in 13 x 9-inch baking pan. Drizzle with 1
Tablespoon olive oil; stir to coat. Roast at 375°F for 35 to 40 minutes or
until tender.

Meanwhile, soak raisins in hot water for 5 minutes. Drain and set aside.

In large bowl, combine balsamic vinegar, honey, olive oil, basil and
oregano; whisk until blended. Add roasted peppers and raisins; toss
lightly to coat. Serve at room temperature.

Serving Suggestions

**Flavor is best when served at room temperature. If
made ahead, cover and refrigerate salad. Bring to room
temperature before serving.**

Sweet & Spicy Avocados

Makes 6 servings

ingredients

1/4 cup butter
1/4 cup honey
1/4 cup catsup
2 Tablespoons cider vinegar
2 teaspoons Worcestershire sauce
A few drops hot pepper sauce
2 avocados
Fresh orange and pink grapefruit slices, optional
Fresh cilantro or herbs, optional

directions

Combine butter, honey, catsup, vinegar, Worcestershire and pepper sauce in small saucepan and heat, stirring until smooth. Keep warm. Halve, seed and skin avocados. Place cut-sides down on board and slice crosswise into crescents. Overlap slices on appetizer plates. Add orange and grapefruit slices to plates if desired. Drizzle 2 Tablespoons warmed sauce over each plate, allowing it to pool underneath avocado.

Add a sprig of cilantro or fresh herb to each plate if desired.

Snacks

Apple Snacksters with Honey & Peanut Butter

Makes 4 servings

ingredients

3/4 cup chunky peanut butter
1/3 cup honey
4 large Granny Smith or Red Delicious apples, stems removed
4 small sprigs fresh mint, optional
Cold water
An adult to help with slicing the apples

directions

1. In a small bowl, mix peanut butter and honey together until well blended. Set aside.
2. Fill a large bowl with cold water and stir in lemon juice. Set aside.
3. For each apple, choose a type of Snackster below and follow the steps. You might want to ask an adult to help cut up the apples.

To Make a Snackster Stacker

1. Use an apple corer to remove the center of the apple, making a hollow space from stem end through the bottom.
2. With a sharp knife, cut apple crosswise into 4 thick slices.
3. Dip apple slices in lemon water and gently pat dry with paper towels.
4. Starting with the bottom piece, use a butter knife to spread the peanut butter mixture on the cut sides of each slice and gently press them together to reassemble the apple.
5. To make a stem, top apple with a mint sprig.

To Make a Snackster Dipper

1. With a sharp knife, cut each apple in half from stem end to bottom.
2. Cut each half into 4 to 6 wedges. With knife or melon ballet remove apple core from each wedge.
3. Dip wedges in lemon water and gently pat dry with paper towels.
4. Spoon the peanut butter mixture into a small bowl and surround with apple wedges for dipping.

Choc "oat" late-Honey "Smash" Snacks

Makes 4 dozen

ingredients

2-1/2 cups thin pretzel sticks, broken into 1-inch pieces
2-1/4 cups Quaker© oats
(quick-cooking or old fashioned), uncooked
1 cup raisins
1 cup dry roasted peanuts, optional
1 package (10 oz.) peanut butter-flavored chips
2 cups semi-sweet chocolate chips
3/4 cup honey

directions

In large bowl, combine pretzels, oats, raisins and, if desired, peanuts; mix well. In large saucepan, combine peanut butter-flavored chips, chocolate chips and honey; heat over low heat, stirring constantly, until chips are melted.

Immediately pour over oat mixture, stirring until all dry ingredients are coated with chocolate mixture. Spread and "smash" mixture onto foil-lined cookie sheet, working the mixture to the edges of the sheet (mixture will be 3/8- to 1/2-inch thick depending upon size of cookie sheet). Place in refrigerator until firm. Break into pieces. Store tightly covered at room temperature.

Cook's Tip: Substitute 1 package (11 oz.) butterscotch-flavored chips for peanut butter-flavored chips.

Chocolate Date Bars

Makes 24 servings

ingredients

1-1/4 cups hot water
8 oz. chopped pitted dates
1-1/4 teaspoon baking soda
3/4 cup honey
1/4 cup soft butter or margarine
2 eggs
1-1/4 cups flour
1/2 teaspoon salt
1 teaspoon vanilla
1/2 cup rolled oats
12 oz. mini chocolate pieces
1 cup chopped nuts

directions

Simmer water, dates and one teaspoon soda together in saucepan for 10 minutes. Set aside to cool. In large mixing bowl, cream honey with butter until fluffy. Add eggs, one at a time, beating well after each addition. Sift together flour, salt and 1/4 teaspoon soda. Blend into creamed mixture. Stir in dates and liquid, vanilla, rolled oats and one half chocolate pieces. Spread batter into greased 9x13-inch baking pan. Sprinkle remaining chocolate pieces and nuts over top. Bake at 350°F 35 minutes. Cool before cutting into bars.

Dessert Variation: Serve warm, cut into squares. Top with soft vanilla ice cream or honey sweetened whipped cream.

Honey Granola Squares

Makes 9 servings

ingredients

3 cups low-fat granola
3/4 cup dried fruit (apples, apricots, cherries, cranberries or pears),
finely chopped
1/2 cup honey
1/4 cup vegetable oil
3/4 teaspoon vanilla extract
3 egg whites, lightly beaten

directions

In a large bowl, mix together granola and dried fruit. In a small saucepan,
heat honey, oil and vanilla over medium heat, stirring until honey is dissolved. Pour honey mixture over granola and mix until thoroughly coated.
Pour egg whites over granola mixture; mix well. Pack mixture firmly into
an 8-inch square nonstick baking pan. Bake at 325°F for 40 minutes or
until deep golden brown. Place pan on a cooling rack; cool completely
before cutting into squares, approximately 2-1/2-inches each.

Honey Glazed Popcorn

Makes 2 cups

ingredients

3/4 cup butter or margarine
2/3 cup honey
2/3 cup packed brown sugar
1/2 teaspoon ground cinnamon
1/4 teaspoon salt
2-1/2 teaspoons vanilla
1/2 teaspoon baking soda
3 quarts popped popcorn
1-1/2 cups roasted peanuts

directions

Melt butter in large saucepan; stir in honey, sugar, cinnamon and salt. Bring to boil; stir constantly. Reduce heat to medium; boil without stirring for 5 minutes. Remove from heat; quickly stir in vanilla and soda.

Place popcorn in large, heat-proof bowl; slowly pour syrup over popcorn while stirring. Add peanuts; mix thoroughly.

Pour into 2 greased 15-1/4 x 10-1/4x3/4-inch baking pans. Bake at 250°F for 45 minutes; stir every 15 minutes with spatula, being certain to scrape honey mixture from pan and coat popcorn thoroughly each time. Remove from oven; cool.

Break into serving-sized pieces. Store in tightly covered container.

Honey Spiced Nuts

Makes 3 cups

ingredients

1/2 cup honey
2 Tablespoons butter, divided
1/2 teaspoon grated orange peel
1/2 teaspoon ground cinnamon
3 cups raw nuts, (walnuts, pecans, cashews, almonds, etc.)

directions

Stovetop Method:

In heavy pan, combine honey, butter, orange peel, and cinnamon. Heat to boiling over medium-high heat, stirring constantly. Reduce heat to medium and cook to 235°F. Stir in nuts, and continue to stir 4 to 5 minutes more, until nuts are glazed. Pour onto parchment paper or buttered foil and spread into a single layer to cool.

Oven Method:

Preheat oven to 325°F. Line a 13 x 9 x 2-inch pan with foil. Tear another sheet of foil the same size and place on counter; butter both. Pour nuts into pan; set aside. In a microwave-safe, 1-cup measure, combine honey, 2 Tablespoons butter, orange peel, and cinnamon. Microwave 60 to 90 seconds, stirring occasionally, until butter is melted. Pour honey mixture over nuts and stir until all are coated. Bake for 20 minutes, stirring every 5 minutes. Remove from oven and pour onto reserved buttered foil, spreading nuts into a single layer to cool. Store in airtight container.

Nutty Honey-Banana Cupcakes

Makes 12 servings

ingredients

1-1/4 cups all-purpose flour
1/4 cup wheat germ
1 teaspoon baking powder
1 teaspoon ground cinnamon
1/4 teaspoon baking soda
1/4 teaspoon salt
1/4 cup butter or margarine, softened
2/3 cup honey
1 large egg
1 teaspoon vanilla
3 Tablespoons milk
1 medium ripe banana, mashed or pureed (1/2 cup puree)
1/2 cup chopped pecans or almonds, optional

directions

Preheat oven to 350°F. Spray muffin cup pans with cooking spray. Stir together flour, wheat germ, baking powder, cinnamon, soda and salt, in large bowl. Set aside. Beat butter on medium speed until light. Beat in honey until mixture is blended. Beat in egg, vanilla, milk and mashed banana until blended. Beat in flour mixture on low speed of mixer until well blended. Spoon batter into prepared muffin cups about 2/3 full. Bake 20 to 25 minutes, or until wooden pick inserted in center comes out clean. Cool pan on wire rack.

Peanut Butter Toasties

Makes 8 servings

ingredients

1-1/4 cups granola with raisins
1/4 cup creamy peanut butter
2 slices whole grain bread
1/3 cup honey

directions

Mix granola, honey, peanut butter and a pinch of salt in a medium bowl.

Toast bread in toaster oven. Remove toast from oven and spread a generous amount of the granola mixture to cover completely.

Return to toaster oven and bake 3 minutes at 350°F until mixture softens. Cut into quarters and serve warm or at room temperature.

Pineapple Orange Honey Smoothie

Makes 5 (8-ounce) servings

ingredients

1 cup milk
1-1/2 cups pineapple, diced
1 cup plain yogurt
1/3 cup pure honey
2 Tablespoons orange juice
1 teaspoon orange zest
5 to 10 ice cubes, optional

directions

In a blender, combine all ingredients except ice cubes and blend until smooth. If desired, add ice cubes, one at a time, and blend until smooth.

Pack-Along Snack Bars

Makes 48 servings

ingredients

4 cups rolled oats
1 cup flaked coconut
1 cup wheat germ
1 cup almonds, chopped
1 teaspoon cinnamon
1 teaspoon salt
1/2 cup vegetable oil
1 cup honey
1 teaspoon vanilla

directions

In a 9x13-inch pan combine oats, coconut, wheat germ, nuts, cinnamon and salt. Set aside. In a bowl, blend together oil, honey and vanilla. Pour over dry ingredients and mix until well coated. Bake at 350°F 25 to 30 minutes, stirring four times during baking. Press hot mixture into a greased 10x15-inch jelly roll pan using a rolling pin. Cool and cut into 48 bars.

Microwave Method:

Microwave granola mixture on HIGH 10 to 12 minutes, stirring every 4 minutes until toasted. Continue as above.

Scorin' Honey S'mores

Makes 6 servings

ingredients

12 cinnamon or chocolate flavored graham crackers,
2x2-inch squares
2 Tablespoons smooth peanut butter
2 Tablespoons honey
1 medium ripe banana, sliced

directions

Arrange six graham crackers on serving plate. Stir together peanut butter and honey until blended. Spread peanut butter mixture generously over six crackers. Arrange banana slices over peanut butter. Place second graham cracker on top of each.

Side Dishes

Balsamic Onions with Honey

Makes 6 servings

ingredients

3 large red onions (about 3 lbs.)
1 Tablespoon + 1/4 cup water
6 Tablespoons honey
1/4 cup balsamic vinegar or red wine vinegar
3 Tablespoons butter or margarine, melted
1 teaspoon paprika
1 teaspoon ground coriander
1/2 teaspoon salt
1/8 teaspoon ground red pepper

directions

Peel onions and cut crosswise into halves. Place cut-side down in shallow baking dish just large enough to hold onions in single layer. Sprinkle with 1 tablespoon water; cover with foil. Bake at 350°F 30 minutes.

Combine honey, vinegar, remaining 1/4 cup water, butter, paprika, coriander, salt and red pepper in small bowl.

Remove onions from oven and turn cut side up. Spoon half of honey mixture over onions. Bake, uncovered, 15 minutes more.

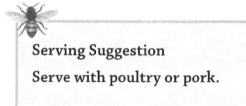

Serving Suggestion

Serve with poultry or pork.

California Two-Bean Salad

Makes 8 servings

ingredients

1/2 lb. dry blackeye beans, cooked
1 red onion, chopped
1 stalk celery, minced
1/2 green bell pepper, minced
1 dill pickle, chopped
2 sprigs parsley, minced
1 can (16 oz.) red kidney beans, drained and rinsed
1 jar (6 oz.) marinated artichoke hearts
1/3 cup salad oil
2 Tablespoons honey
2 teaspoons oregano
1 Tablespoon Dijon mustard
1 teaspoon salt
1 teaspoon coarsely ground black pepper

directions

Soak and cook beans according to package directions. Drain thoroughly.
While still hot, combine with onion, celery, green pepper, pickle, parsley
and kidney beans. Drain marinade from artichoke hearts and combine
with oil, honey, oregano, mustard, and 1 teaspoon each salt and pepper.
Pour over bean mixture, tossing lightly. Add artichoke hearts. Cover and
chill 24 hours. Taste and add more salt as needed.

Grilled Corn with Spiced Honey Butter

Makes 8 servings

ingredients

1/2 cup butter, softened
1/3 cup honey
1 tsp. chili powder
8 ears fresh corn
8 lime wedges
1/4 cup fresh cilantro, chopped

directions

In a small bowl stir together the butter, honey and chili powder; set aside. Fold back husks and remove silk from corn; pull husks back up over corn. Place corn in a large bowl of ice water and soak for 15 minutes. Remove and shake off excess water. Place on grill over medium hot coals and cook for 15 to 20 minutes, turning frequently. Remove husks and spread each ear with seasoned butter. Sprinkle with cilantro and serve with lime wedges.

Honey Baked Beans

Makes 4 to 6 servings

ingredients

4 slices bacon, diced
1/2 cup chopped onion
4-1/2 cups cooked navy beans*
1/2 cup honey
1/2 cup ketchup
1 Tablespoon prepared mustard
1 Tablespoon Worcestershire sauce

directions

Sauté bacon and onion until onion is tender; combine with remaining ingredients in shallow 2-quart oven-safe baking dish. Cover with lid or aluminum foil and bake at 350°F 30 minutes. Uncover and bake 45 minutes longer.

Three 15 oz. cans cooked navy beans can be substituted.

Honey Corn Cakes

Makes 12 to 14 corn cakes

ingredients

1/4 cup honey
2 cans (15.25 oz. each) corn kernels, drained
3 eggs
1 cup flour
1/2 cup Milk
1/2 teaspoon garlic salt

directions

Combine all ingredients. Heat skillet lightly coated with olive oil to medium temperature. Pour 1/3-cup portions of corn cake mix into skillet and cook for about 1-1/2 to 2 minutes on each side.

Honey Nut Squash

Makes 4 servings

ingredients

2 acorn squash
4 Tablespoons honey
2 Tablespoons chopped walnuts
2 Tablespoons seedless raisins
2 Tablespoons margarine, melted
2 Tablespoons Worcestershire sauce

directions

Cut acorn squash lengthwise into halves; do not remove seeds. Place cut side up in baking pan or on baking sheet. Bake at 400°F 30 to 45 minutes or until soft. Remove seeds and fibers.

Combine honey, butter, walnuts, raisins and Worcestershire sauce; spoon into squash. Bake 5 to 10 minutes more until lightly glazed.

Microwave Method:

Cut acorn squash lengthwise into halves and remove seeds. Microwave according to manufacturer's directions. Combine honey, butter, walnuts, raisins and Worcestershire sauce; spoon into squash. Microwave at HIGH (100%) 30 seconds or until thoroughly heated and lightly glazed.

Raw Fresh Applesauce

Makes 1-1/2 cups

ingredients

3 apples, pared, cored and diced
1/4 cup honey
1/4 cup apple juice, orange juice or pineapple juice

directions

Place all ingredients in blender or food processor. Puree to desired smoothness.

Red-Skin Potato Salad with Honey Dill Dressing

Makes 6 servings

ingredients

1-1/2 lbs. small red new potatoes
4 strips bacon
1 medium onion, diced
6 Tablespoons honey
6 Tablespoons apple cider vinegar
1/2 teaspoon cornstarch
1/2 teaspoon water
2 Tablespoons chopped fresh dill or 1 Tablespoon dried dill
1 bunch watercress, washed and chopped

directions

In large pot, boil whole potatoes in salted water until; tender but firm. Drain and cool. While potatoes are cooling, sauté bacon until crisp in large frying pan. Remove bacon and set aside. Add onion to bacon drippings; cooking until soft, about 3 minutes. Add honey and vinegar to pan; stir to combine and bring to a boil. Blend cornstarch with water; stir into honey mixture. Cook until mixture thickens. Remove from heat. Crumble bacon; stir bacon and dill into dressing. Cut cooled potatoes in half, leaving skins on. In large bowl, combine potatoes and watercress. Pour dressing over salad and toss gently. Serve immediately.

Stir-Fried Zucchini and Carrots

Makes 4 servings

ingredients

1 Tablespoon vegetable oil
3 medium-sized carrots, julienned
3 medium-sized zucchini, julienned
1 small onion, vertically sliced
2 Tablespoons honey
1-1/2 teaspoons lemon juice
1/2 teaspoon fresh lemon peel, grated
Salt and pepper, to taste

directions

Add oil to hot skillet; add carrots, zucchini and onion and stir-fry until vegetables are crisp-tender. Stir in remaining ingredients and cook 1 minute longer.

Wild Rice & Mushroom Stuffing

Makes 4 servings

ingredients

1 cup wild rice
4 cups water, salted to taste
1 Tablespoon oil
1/2 cup minced onion
1/2 cup chopped celery
1 teaspoon minced garlic
2 cups sliced mushrooms
1/4 cup chopped dried apricots
2 Tablespoons minced parsley
1/4 cup honey

directions

In small saucepan, combine wild rice with salted water. Bring to a boil. Cover, reduce heat and simmer until tender, approximately 45 minutes. While rice is cooking, heat oil in skillet over medium-high heat. Stir in onions, celery and garlic; sauté until onion is translucent and celery is soft, about 7 minutes. Add mushrooms; sauté until mushrooms are soft, about 3 minutes. Remove pan from heat. When rice is cooked, drain in a colander. In large bowl, combine rice and mushroom-onion mixture. Add apricots, parsley and honey, stirring until mixed well. Serve warm as a side dish or use to stuff poultry.

Desserts

Apple Honey Crisp with Warm Nutmeg Cream

Makes 6 servings

ingredients

2 lbs. apples, quartered and sliced (1-1/2 quarts)
1/2 cup plus 1/4 cup honey, (separated)
1 teaspoon cinnamon
1/2 teaspoon nutmeg
1 cup flour
1/4 cup butter, softened
Warm Nutmeg Cream, (recipe follows) or ice cream

directions

Toss apples with 1/2 cup honey, cinnamon and nutmeg in bowl. Turn into 2-quart baking dish. For topping, beat flour with butter and 1/4 cup honey until crumbly; sprinkle over apples. Bake at 350°F for 40 to 45 minutes or until apples are tender and topping is golden. Serve with Warm Nutmeg Cream or ice cream.

Warm Nutmeg Cream

Makes 1/2 cup

ingredients

1/2 cup whipping cream
2 Tablespoons honey
2 Tablespoons butter
1/4 teaspoon nutmeg

directions

Combine all ingredients in saucepan and bring to boil. Simmer, stirring often, for 5 minutes or until mixture thickens slightly.

Apricot Honey Oat Bar Cookies

Makes 8 servings

ingredients

1-1/2 cups old-fashioned rolled oats, uncooked
1/2 cup finely chopped dried apricots
1/2 cup honey
1/4 cup nonfat plain yogurt
2 egg whites
2 Tablespoons wheat germ
2 Tablespoons all-purpose flour
3 Tablespoons butter or margarine, melted
1/2 teaspoon ground cinnamon
1/2 teaspoon vanilla
1/4 teaspoon salt

directions

Spray 8-inch square baking pan with nonstick cooking spray. Combine all ingredients in large bowl; mix well. Spread mixture evenly into prepared pan. Bake at 325°F about 25 minutes or until center is firm and edges are lightly browned. Cool and cut into 2-inch squares.

Banana Fritters with Honey Cream

Makes 8 servings

ingredients

4 medium bananas, firm but ripe
1/2 cup heavy cream
2 eggs
2 teaspoons sugar
1 cup corn flake crumbs
1/3 cup olive oil
Honey Cream

directions

Peel bananas. Halve lengthwise and crosswise. Set aside. In shallow bowl whisk cream, egg and sugar. Coat bananas in cream mixture, then in crumbs. In a 12-inch skillet heat oil over medium heat. Sauté fritters about 2 minutes per side until crisp and golden. Serve with Honey Cream.

Honey Cream

ingredients

1 cup dairy sour cream
1 cup plain yogurt
1/2 cup honey
1/2 teaspoon vanilla extract

directions

In a small bowl stir all ingredients. Refrigerate until serving.

Bee Nutty Choco-Chip Cookies

Makes 16 servings

ingredients

1/2 cup honey
1/2 cup peanut butter
1/2 cup butter or margarine
1/4 cup packed brown sugar
1 egg
1-1/2 teaspoon vanilla
2 cups flour
1/2 teaspoon baking soda
1/2 teaspoon salt
6 oz. chocolate morsels
1/2 cup roasted peanuts, coarsely chopped

directions

Combine honey, peanut butter, butter and brown sugar in a large
bowl; beat until light and fluffy. Add egg and vanilla; mix thoroughly.
Combine flour, soda and salt; mix well. Stir into peanut butter mixture.
Stir in chocolate morsels and peanuts. Using a 1/4 cup measure for each
cookie, drop onto ungreased cookie sheet; flatten slightly. Bake at 350°F
8 to 10 minutes or until lightly browned. Remove to rack and cool.

Carrot Spice Cake

Makes 10 to 12 servings

ingredients

1/2 cup butter or margarine
1 cup honey
2 eggs
2 cups finely grated carrots
1/2 cup golden raisins
1/2 cup chopped nuts
1/4 cup orange juice
2 teaspoons vanilla
1 cup whole wheat flour
1 cup unbleached flour
2 teaspoons baking powder
1-1/2 teaspoons ground cinnamon
1 teaspoon baking soda
1/2 teaspoon salt
1/2 teaspoon ground ginger
1/4 Tablespoon ground nutmeg

directions

In large mixing bowl, cream butter until fluffy. Beat in honey in fine stream until well blended. Add eggs one at a time, beating well after each addition. In small bowl, combine carrots, raisins, nuts, orange juice and vanilla, set aside. Combine dry ingredients; set aside. Add dry ingredients to creamed mixture alternately with carrot mixture, beginning and ending with dry ingredients. Turn batter into greased 12x8x2-inch pan.

Bake at 350°F 35 to 45 minutes or until wooden pick inserted near center comes out clean. Cool in pan 10 minutes. Turn onto wire cake rack.

Fudgy Honey Brownies with Honey Whipped Cream

Makes 8 servings

ingredients

1 package (19 3/4 oz.) fudge brownie mix
1/3 cup vegetable oil
1/4 cup water
2 Tablespoons honey
1 egg
Honey Whipped Cream
Bottled hot fudge topping

directions

Combine all ingredients; mix and spread in greased and floured 5-cup heart-shaped baking pan*. Bake according to package directions for 8x8-inch pan. Cool thoroughly. Invert onto serving plate. Spread with Honey Whipped Cream or pipe cream through pastry tube. Drizzle with hot fudge topping.

*An 8x8x2-inch pan can be substituted

Honey Whipped Cream

Makes 2 cups

ingredients

1 cup whipping cream
3 Tablespoons honey
1 teaspoon vanilla

directions

Beat whipping cream until mixture thickens; gradually add honey and beat until soft peaks form. Fold in vanilla.

Honey Almond Biscotti

Makes 3 dozen

ingredients

1/2 cup butter or margarine, softened
3/4 cup honey
2 eggs
1 teaspoon vanilla extract
3-1/2 cups all-purpose flour
2 teaspoons anise seeds
2 teaspoons ground cinnamon
1/2 teaspoon baking powder
1/2 teaspoon salt
1/4 teaspoon baking soda
1 cup dried cranberries
3/4 cup slivered almonds

directions

Using electric mixer, beat butter until light; gradually add honey, eggs and vanilla, beating until smooth. In small bowl, combine flour, aniseseeds, cinnamon, baking powder, salt and baking soda; gradually add to honey mixture, mixing well. Stir in cranberries and almonds.

Shape dough into two 10x3x1-inch logs on greased baking sheet. Bake at 350°F for 20 minutes or until light golden brown. Remove from oven to wire rack; cool 5 minutes. Reduce oven to 300°F. Transfer logs to cutting board. Cut each log into 1/2-inch slices; arrange on baking sheet. Bake 20 minutes or until crisp. Cool on wire racks.

Honey Lemon Cheesecake

Makes 12 servings

ingredients

1-1/2 cups broken vanilla wafer cookies
1/2 cup slivered almonds, toasted
1/4 cup butter or margarine, melted
11 oz. cream cheese
1-1/2 cups milk, divided
1/4 cup fresh lemon juice
2 teaspoons freshly grated lemon peel
1 envelope unflavored gelatin
1/2 cup honey (Orange Blossom, Sage or Tupelo)

directions

Place cookies and nuts in blender or food processor container; process until coarse crumbs. Add melted butter; process until blended. Pour crumb mixture into 9-inch spring form pan; spread and press evenly onto bottom and up sides of pan to form crust. Freeze while preparing filling.

Using electric mixer, beat cream cheese until smooth. Slowly add 1 1/4 cups milk, mixing until smooth and well blended. Beat in lemon juice and peel; set aside. In small saucepan, sprinkle gelatin over remaining 1/4 cup milk; let stand 1 minute. Stir over low heat until gelatin is completely dissolved. Stir in honey; whisk to blend. Add to cheese mixture, mixing until well blended. Freeze 15 minutes then whisk partially set cheesecake mixture until smooth. Pour into prepared crust and refrigerate at least 2 hours.

Drizzle with honey and serve with fresh fruits and Honey Whipped Cream, if desired.

Topping ideas: fresh fruits, such as raspberries, blueberries, strawberries, Honey Whipped Cream

Honey Strawberry Tart

Makes 8 servings

ingredients

1/3 cup honey
1 Tablespoon lemon juice
1 baked or ready-to-eat 9-inch pie shell
4 cups halved fresh strawberries
Mint sprigs, for garnish, optional

directions

Combine honey and lemon juice in small bowl; mix well. Brush bottom of pie shell with mixture. Fill shell with strawberries. Drizzle remaining honey mixture over berries. Garnish with mint sprigs, if desired.

Tip:

Prepare honey glaze and strawberries. Fill shell and glaze strawberries just before serving to prevent shell from becoming soggy.

Triple Chocolate Honey Fudge

Makes 64 servings

ingredients

1-1/3 cups granulated sugar
1 jar (8 oz.) marshmallow cream
2/3 cup evaporated milk
1/4 cup honey
1/4 cup butter or margarine
1/4 teaspoon salt
2 cups semi-sweet chocolate chips
1/2 cup milk chocolate chips
1-1/2 teaspoons vanilla extract
1/2 cup toasted nuts, chopped
1/2 cup white chocolate chips

directions

Spray an 8x8-inch pan with nonstick cooking spray; set aside. In medium saucepan, combine sugar, marshmallow cream, milk, honey, butter and salt. Bring to a boil; stir occasionally. Boil for 5 minutes; stir constantly. Remove from heat and stir in semi-sweet and milk chocolate chips until melted. Stir in nuts and vanilla; pour into pan. Sprinkle with white chocolate chips over top and allow to melt. Using small spatula swirl white chocolate. Cool. Cut into 1-inch pieces.

Upside-Down Peach Berry Pie

Makes 8 servings

ingredients

Crust:

1/3 cup wheat germ

1/4 lb. (1 stick) butter, chilled
and cut into 10 pieces

1 egg

4 cups ripe peaches or nectarines,
peeled and sliced

1/3 cup honey

1 Tablespoon cornstarch

1-1/4 cups all-purpose flour

1 teaspoon freshly grated lemon peel

3 Tablespoons honey

Filling:

2 cups blueberries, raspberries,
blackberries or any combination

2 Tablespoons fresh lemon juice

directions

For pastry, combine flour, wheat germ and lemon peel in a large bowl.
Cut in butter with two knives until mixture resembles coarse crumbs. In
a small bowl, beat honey with egg. Add to dry ingredients all at once;
stir with fork just until dough starts to hold together. Gather dough into
a ball; place on waxed paper or plastic wrap and flatten to 3/4-inch thick
disk. Wrap tightly; chill at least 1 hour or overnight.

Heat oven to 400°F. Remove pastry from refrigerator.

For filling, combine peaches and berries in a large bowl. In a small bowl,
combine honey, lemon juice and cornstarch; mix well. Add to fruit; stir
gently until fruit is evenly coated. Spoon into 11 x 7-inch baking dish.

On a sheet of lightly floured waxed paper, roll pastry into 11x7-inch
rectangle. Cut 6 to 8 slits in rectangle. Invert onto a baking dish;
peel off paper.

Bake 10 minutes. Reduce oven temperature to 350°F. Continue baking
25 to 30 minutes or until fruit is bubbly and pastry is golden brown. If
pastry begins to brown too quickly, cover loosely with foil. Serve warm
or at room temperature.

Honey Health Glossary

Antimicrobial
A substance than can be used to kill or prevent the growth of harmful bacteria without damaging fragile tissue.

The use of honey as a gentle, effective antimicrobial has become even more promising of late, as the emergence of "superbugs" (bacteria resistant to antibiotics) has become more widespread. In many cases involving superbugs, honey has proven to kill bacteria where conventional antibiotics have failed.

Antioxidant
A molecule that slows or stops oxidation, a chemical reaction that can produce free radicals.

Foods high in antioxidants may help prevent cellular damage and protect against the development of numerous diseases. Honey's antioxidant capacities are believed to be the result of several compounds acting together, including phenolics, peptides, organic acids and enzymes.

Beehive
Enclosed structure where honeybees live. There, the queen bee, worker bees, and drone bees live together in a complex, carefully organized community, where each bee has a specific task to perform. For example, the queen bee is the only bee to lay eggs in the hive; she can lay more than 1 million eggs in her lifetime! The hive is made of a honeycomb structure that forms hexagonal "cells." In these cells, the young bees (called pupa) are fed and raised, and   honey is stored.

Hives can be manmade or created by bees themselves.

Beeswax
Another product of nectar secreted by honeybees used to build the beehive. Typically a yellow to grayish-brown color, beeswax is in fact edible, and can also be used to make products like sweet-smelling beeswax candles.

Bifidobacteria
A good form of bacteria found in the colon. Consuming foods that contain prebiotics, such as honey, can increase the presence of bifidobacteria.

Honey
Sweet tasting and golden amber to light auburn in color, honey is produced by bees using flower nectar. To produce honey, bees consume, and then regurgitate flower nectar until it obtains the proper consistency.

Honey is stored in the hexagonal "cells" of the hive. During the winter months, when nectar and pollen from flowers are not available to eat, bees subsist on the stored honey.

As a food product, honey is made up mostly of fructose, glucose and water, but also contains a variety of other sugars and trace amounts of enzymes, mineral and vitamins.

Honeycomb
The pattern of hexagonal cells that make up the beeswax. These cells hold the queen bee's eggs as well as stored food. To harvest honey this comb is removed, emptied and then typically returned.

Infant Botulism
Bacterial infection caused by spores that are found throughout our environment and in soil, dust, air and in raw fruits and vegetables. Adults and children can consume these spores with no problems. Infants however lack a fully developed gastrointestinal tract, allowing these spores to cause botulism. For this reason, honey shouldn't be fed to infants under one year of age.

Nectar
Sugar-rich liquid secreted by flowering plants. Nectar is harvested and brought back to the hive by honeybees. There, the nectar is eaten and used to produce beeswax and food in the form of honey, which is stored in the hive.

Pollination
Process that takes place when honeybees, traveling from flower to flower to gather pollen and nectar, transfer pollen on their bodies from one plant to another. This facilitates plant fertilization and reproduction.

Spinner
A machine used to extract the honey from the harvested honeycomb. The honeycomb is placed in the center of a machine and rotated, so as to draw the honey out of the comb and collect in the basin of the spinner.

Superbugs
Illnesses caused by strains of bacteria that are resistant to antibiotics.

FAQ

Honey Properties

Why does one type of honey taste or look different from other kinds?
The taste and color or honey varies widely depending on what type of flower the bee visited for the nectar to make the honey. Try a number of honeys, pick your favorites, and enjoy them on their own or in a selection of recipes.

What is "raw honey"?
There is no official definition for "raw" honey, but it usually means honey that has not been heated or filtered.

You may have heard the term "raw food," which is a method of eating fresh fruit and vegetables uncooked in order to reap the most nutritional benefits from a vegetable or a fruit. Although "eating raw" in this manner may have its benefits, "raw honey" is not generally more healthy than other types of honey.

Does honey expire or go bad?
Over time, and depending on the temperature at which honey is stored, chemical changes can occur in honey and it can darken and lose its intensity of flavor or crystallize. For these reasons, it is best to enjoy honey within two years of purchase.

My honey has crystallized/become solid. Can I still eat it?
Yes! Crystallization is a natural process during which the sugar in honey (glucose) separates from the liquid honey.

If your honey crystallizes, place the jar in a pot of warm water and stir until the crystals dissolve. Be careful not to burn the honey or boil it.

You can eat honey in its crystallized form if you like. It works great spread over toast or dropped into hot tea!

Bees and Beekeeping

How do bees pollinate plants?

As bees fly from flower to flower in search of nectar, they brush against the pollen-bearing parts of a flower. When they fly to another flower, they bring with them the pollen from the other plant. This process pollinates the flowers, allowing many types of plants, including a great deal of our food crops, to reproduce and grow in abundance.

Almonds, apples, avocados, blueberries, cantaloupes, cherries, cranberries, cucumbers, sunflowers, watermelon are just some of the foods we eat that need help from the honeybees to be pollinated so they can grow in abundance.

How do bees make honey?

Honey is the sweet, golden colored liquid produced by bees from the nectar of flowers. When a worker bee returns to the hive with nectar, the bee adds enzymes to the nectar which reduce the moisture content in the nectar and, by this process, create honey.

Bees also produce the edible wax that makes up the hive's honeycomb pattern. The honey is stored in the hexogen shaped "cells" of the hive's walls. When all the cells have been filled with honey, the bees top off the cells with a wax "cap." When the honey is harvested, the beekeeper extracts the honey from these cells of the beehive.

Threats to the Bee Population

To understand the impacts of colony collapse disorder, the true threats to the bee population must first be recognized. While the application of chemicals, including insecticides, pesticides and miticides, have helped lawns, crops and gardens to thrive, these chemicals are slowly destroying other elements of the ecosystem. Leaching into the water and soil systems, these substances are proving to be a growing threat to the health and safety of bee populations. Specifically, miticides are commonly used by commercial beekeepers in controlling varroa mites in their bee populations. Consequently, trace quantities are found in the wax sheets produced from the excess wax of the miticide treated hives. Made and sold by bee keeping supply companies, beekeepers purchase wax foundation sheets, unaware of the possible transfer of chemical content.

Global warming has posed another serious danger to bee communities. During those surprisingly warmer winter days, bees are easily coaxed out of their semi-hibernation and begin foraging for early pollen sources, further depleting honey stores used for energy. Furthermore, warmer winter temperatures give mites an early start on breeding, allowing them to have a much stronger presence in the springtime.

Monoculture pollination has been an increasing problem as well. Pollination of a single crop has forced bees to survive on a limited diet deficient in nutrients. A similar problem is seen in the controlled reproduction of bees. Select breeding with honey production in mind has reduced the once diverse gene pool. Looking to breed the best producers, farmers have reduced the gene pool, likely creating strains of bees that have more difficulty in naturally fighting off infection. The treatment of infections with antibiotics has been successful in the short run. However, these treatments only proliferate future bees' ability to naturally fight parasites and infections.

Further problems with bee health have arisen as a result of genetically modified crops. Not only can bees easily spread pollen from genetically modified crops to non-genetically modified crops, they've also been subjected to the BT toxin & I.M.D., a neonicotinoid engineered as an insecticide for the genetically modified crops. These toxins are easily ingested when any part of the crop is consumed, which includes the pollen. As a result, bees have been shown to have certain defects, including loss of navigation and homing skills and shorter life spans. In addition to all these threats, beekeepers transporting hives for agricultural pollination have seen combating stress as a growing problem. Along with the causes mentioned above, the long-distance transport of hives by tractor trailers has further stressed the bees' already weakened systems.

Helen Faraday-Young is producer and coordinator of Bee Native, a non-profit organization dedicated to strengthening the honeybee population through education, training, and research.

Resources

National Honey Board

Visit the website for more recipes, as well as more information on honey and health. You can also sign up for the monthly newsletter, "Honey Buzz," to receive the latest honey news as well as delicious seasonal recipes.
www.honey.com

HoneyLocator.com

This website, sponsored by the National Honey Board, provides all the information you need to "find the honey you're looking for." Visit this site for details on honey varieties as well as information on where to find certain types of honey.
www.honeylocator.com

Bee Native

Visit the website below for more information about bees and the current threats to the bee population. Learn what you can do to help.
www.beenative.org

Local Harvest

This site can help you find farms near you so you can order honey locally. Finding honey near where you live is a great way to support local farmers and help save the earth—the less distance between you and any product, the less pollution is produced during transportation!
www.localharvest.org

Also in the *Cooking Well* series...

Cooking Well: Osteoporosis

Cooking Well: Multiple Sclerosis

Cooking Well: Mediterranean

Cooking Well: Wheat Allergies

Cooking Well: Beautiful Skin

Cooking Well: Diabetes

Available at bookstores everywhere